TOTAL FITNESS AFTER 40

THE 7 LIFE CHANGING FOUNDATIONS YOU NEED FOR STRENGTH, HEALTH AND MOTIVATION IN YOUR 40S, 50S, 60S AND BEYOND

NICK SWETTENHAM

WWW.NICKSWETTENHAMFITNESS.COM

CONTENTS

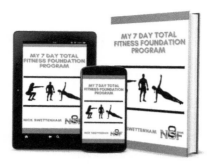

A Special Gift For My Readers

Included with the purchase of this book is My 7 Day Total
Fitness Foundation Program to help you get started on your
fitness journey. This program is a great way to start or adapt
your training using all my 7 foundations.
Click the link below and let us know which email address you
would like it delivered to.

www.nickswettenhamfitness.com

INTRODUCTION

Help! Get me out of this body!

What's happening to me?

This is not what I signed up for.

If you've ever had those thoughts while standing naked in front of a mirror, you're hardly alone. The sad reality is that most people who are in their 40s, 50s and beyond are dissatisfied with their physical condition. Many of them are overweight, under-strength and overwhelmed by aches and pains, chronic illness and plummeting energy levels.

In short, they are pretty pathetic imitations of what they used to be - and of what they should be.

If that's you, you need to know that growing weaker and less fit does not have to be your destiny as you age. You have it within your capacity to wake up every morning better, healthier and stronger than when you went to bed the night before. And that is true whether you're 27, 47, or 67.

Chronologically, age means nothing. In order to preserve your age, you need to preserve your physicality. And the time to start preserving it is now.

That's because, by the time you enter into your fourth decade, your body is beginning to show signs of wear and tear...

- Blood vessels lose their elasticity, making the heart work harder to pump blood around the body
- Muscles, joints and tendons lose strength and flexibility
- Testosterone production plummets
- The metabolism slows down

Society expects you to start going downhill as a result of these natural consequences of aging. After all, it's what everyone else does, right?

Once they hit 40, they get fat, lethargic, sick and decrepit. Every decade the downward spiral continues - then they die.

Is that the sort of future you want?

It doesn't have to be.

You see, there are a whole lot of people who have totally flipped that script. At 40, 50 and even 60 something they are genuinely in the best shape of their entire lives!

How have they done it?

By rejecting the ridiculously low bar that society has set for them and by learning the truth about fitness, health and well-being over 40.

That truth is what you will learn in this book.

It is encompassed within the 7 foundations that you must incorporate into your life in order to stay strong, lean and healthy at any age.

When you know, understand and apply the 7 foundations you will have the solution to the problems that plague many people in their 40s and beyond...

- Lost muscle and strength
- Decreased mobility and flexibility
- Lost confidence in their ability to train intensely

Your body does change when you age, and in this book, you will discover exactly how it does so. More importantly, though, you will find out precisely how you need to adjust your training to compensate for those changes.

This book will also show you how to infuse your mind with the mental strength to power you through the physical changes that will make you more powerful. By applying the strategies I'm about to share with you, you'll become laser-like in your ability to set, hone in on and systematically work toward the accomplishment of your goals.

Critically, we also demystify the whole subject of fitness nutrition. No other subject has led to such confusion, frustration and disappointment. Yet, what you eat is more important than anything else that you do. In Chapter Nine, you will finally learn how to eat the right way for your body.

Of course, there are literally thousands of books on getting in shape. So, why should you listen to what I've got to say?

Well, the honest answer is that you shouldn't. You should listen to the science of fitness, anatomy, biomechanics, kinesiology and nutrition. The great thing about science is that it is objective - it is not swayed by emotion, popularity, gimmicks or money making trends. All of that science is presented, disseminated and distilled in the chapters that follow. In fact, they form the basis of the 7 foundations that will underpin your future fitness program.

The problem with science, however, is that it is often presented by people who have no practical, on the ground experience in the discipline that it is applied to. And that's where I come in. You see, I am a personal fitness trainer who has used these 7 foundations to help hundreds of men and women over the age of 40 to regain their youthful vigor, transform their bodies and become stronger, more agile and healthier than when they were in their 20s and 30s.

I've written this book because I train people every day who, even before they're 40, are struggling with all 7 of these foundations. In the over 40 age-group, though, it is particularly challenging due to changes occurring in their bodies. I find that my clients have little to no knowledge of what is happening, and have either lost their confidence or have never gained it in the first place. I want this book to inspire people to take charge and start implementing these foundations into their workout routines.

I'm passionate about the health and fitness industry – it is a huge part of my life (both work and personal) and I love to help my clients improve their function and quality of life.

Are you ready to show the world, and yourself, that over 40 doesn't have to mean over the hill?

Great, let's get started!

1

AS WE AGE, WE CHANGE

WHAT'S HAPPENING TO MY BODY?

Over the past hundred years there has been a dramatic lengthening of the average human lifespan. For hundreds of years that average hovered around the 35 year mark. By 1900 it was up to around 50. Yet, between 1900 and 2000, it shot up to around 80. Currently the average life expectancy in the US is 78.99 years. Unfortunately, those extended years have not equated to improved health. In addition to the natural consequences of aging, many people in their 40s and beyond suffer from a range of lifestyle related illnesses that negatively affect their quality of life.

In this chapter, we consider the natural physiological changes that are a part of the aging process. We will then identify how the right type of exercise in conjunction with the 7 foundations of optimum health can counter these effects by keeping us stronger, more flexible, agile, coordinated and injury free as we age.

How Your Body Changes as You Age

Cardiovascular System Changes

As it ages, the heart becomes less efficient at pumping blood around the body. As a result, it has to work harder to keep the same quantity of blood moving around the system. At the same time, the blood vessels become less elastic and fatty deposits may build up on the walls of the arteries. As a result, the arteries become stiffer and blood pressure increases.

Bone Density Changes

From the age of 30 onwards, your bone density (having reached its peak) will begin to deteriorate. From that point onward, the bones will begin to shrink. The loss of density will make the bones weaker and more susceptible to fracture. The aging process also causes the vertebrae between the spinal discs to contract, making a person shorter. In fact, from the age of 40 onward, the average person will lose about half an inch in height every 10 years.

Muscle Changes

From around the age of 30, the natural process of aging results in muscle tissue loss. Both the quantity of muscle tissue and the number of muscle fibers are depleted. Fast twitch fibers deplete more so than slow twitch fibers, with the result that the muscles are slower to contract.

By the time they are 75, the average person will lose 25 percent of the muscle mass they had when they were 30. This muscle loss occurs more quickly in the lower part of the body than the upper part.

The reduction in the number of muscle fibers results in diminishing strength levels. This loss of strength, combined with the reduced balance that is another consequence of aging, may result in increased incidences of falling and losing one's balance.

Running in tandem with age related loss of muscle fibers, there is a corresponding loss of motor neurons. Shockingly, by the age of 60, the average person will have only 50 percent of the number of motor neurons they had when they were 20. These motor neurons are what control and drive muscle fiber activity. When they deplete, the muscle fiber will eventually die off.

The muscular system affects virtually every action that we take, so its weakening has profound effects on all areas of life. Age related muscle decline is known as sarcopenia. Its cumulative effect on body functioning shows difficulty in performing everyday tasks, such as carrying groceries, walking up flights of stairs or opening cans.

Hormonal Changes

We can think of hormones like orchestra conductors in that they control and regulate the myriad actions that are taking place in your body every second. Androgenic hormones are those that regulate male characteristics. The prime androgenic hormone is testosterone. Its main job is to regulate sexual functioning. Secondary functions include controlling muscle mass, strength levels, fat deposits and bone density.

Testosterone is well known as the key muscle building hormone. In fact, there is an out of control anabolic steroid market that allows people to inject synthetic versions of testosterone into their veins in order to get bigger and stronger. In addition to aiding the muscle mass increase, testosterone will also slow down muscle loss.

From around the age of 25, natural testosterone production begins to drop off. This age related testosterone decline speeds up when you enter your 30s, dropping by about 1 percent every decade. That's why it is harder for a guy in his 40s to build muscle than a guy in his 20s.

Even though it is a male sex hormone, testosterone is also important for women. That's because it is converted to estrogen (the female sex hormone) as well as promoting bone health, sex drive and fertility.

Testosterone is not the only hormone that diminishes as we age. Most of them do. Even with those that remain at constant levels, the decreased sensitivity of hormone receptors makes them less potent. In addition to testosterone, the key hormones which decline with age are estrogen, melatonin and growth hormone.

Melatonin is known as the sleep hormone. Its age-related decline is a key contributor to the sleep problems that so many people encounter as they age.

In men, the reduction of growth hormone combines with lower testosterone levels to further impact strength and muscle levels.

In women, the lowering of estrogen production is a direct contributor to menopause. This is characterized by the ending of menstruation. The levels of estrogen will fluctuate markedly in the years prior to and just after the onset of menopause. Bone density will decrease quite markedly after menopause. The onset of menopause is also accompanied by hot flashes.

The average age for the onset of menopause in women in America is 52, though it may commence from 45 years onward. Such lifestyle factors as smoking may cause an earlier onset of menopause.

Reduced levels of estrogen lead to other changes after the onset of menopause. These may include vaginal atrophy which makes sexual intercourse painful, thinning of the urinary tract that may make a woman more susceptible to urinary tract infections, and urinary incontinence. Lowered estrogen levels will also result in lowered levels of collagen and elasticity which reduces the elasticity of the skin.

Lower levels of estrogen will also exacerbate the age related decline in bone density. As a consequence of this, women will lose bone mass by about 5 percent more than men in the five years after the onset of menopause. It then levels off to be about the same rate as men.

Post menopause, women will also experience an increased level of LDL (bad) cholesterol, while the HDL (good) level remains the same. Women are also more prone to fat accumulation around the hips and waist after menopause.

Skin Changes

As we age, our skin becomes less elastic, thinner and drier. Fine wrinkles develop naturally but are made worse by long years of exposure to the sun. The main reason for these changes is the reduction in the levels of the fibrous tissue collagen and the flexible protein elastin. As well as making less of these compounds, aging actually changes their chemical structure so that they become less effective in keeping the skin looking young.

Another effect of aging on the skin is a thinning out of the fat layer directly under the skin. This takes away a layer of protection while also exacerbating the wrinkling effect of aging skin. The thinning of this fat layer also removes a means of insulation so that, as we age, we become less tolerant to the cold. At the same time, the body is less efficient at controlling heat. The number of sweat glands and blood vessels reduces with every passing decade. This makes it harder for heat to be moved from within to without the body. For this reason, older people are more likely to succumb to heatstroke.

A final effect of aging on the skin is that it is less able to absorb Vitamin D from the sun. That is why elderly people are more likely to have a Vitamin D deficiency.

Brain & Nervous System Changes

The brain changes more than any other part of the body as we grow older. From around the age of 30, the brain begins to shrink in size. Some areas of the brain get smaller faster than others. The three areas that are most affected are:

- The prefrontal cortex
- The cerebellum
- The hippocampus

It is interesting to note that these three areas are also the last to develop during adolescence. As a result, scientists have developed the last in, first out theory, by which the last parts of the brain to develop are the first parts to deteriorate.

As we age, the neurons in the brain get smaller in size and retract their dendrites. The number of synapses between the brain cells also diminishes, which has marked effects on brain functioning. Neurogenesis, or the creation of new neurons, also slows down with aging. Chemical messengers, including dopamine and serotonin, also become less frequent as we get older.

As a result of these changes in the brain, our memories become less effective, reflexes are slower, and coordination and balance are negatively impaired.

Urinary Tract Changes

Every decade beyond the age of 30, the kidneys become less effective at doing their job of eliminating waste from the body. Ten percent of people over the age of 65 experience a loss of bladder control. Urinary incontinence is more frequent in women than in men. This may occur as a result of the weakening of the sphincter muscles around the opening of the bladder. In men, it is caused by enlargement of the prostate.

Sleeping Pattern Changes

Contrary to what many people think, you do not need less sleep as you age. The reason that a lot of older people find it hard to get as much sleep as when they were younger is a combination of some of the factors we have already mentioned. This includes a lessening of the body's production of melatonin and a need to urinate more frequently.

Body Composition Changes

The natural loss of muscle tissue that occurs with aging is accompanied by most people with an increase in levels of body fat. A person's metabolism will naturally slow down as they age. This means that, even if they maintain the same caloric intake in their 50s as they did in their 30s, they burn fewer of them for energy and store more of them as body fat. In tandem with this is a general slowing down of activity as we age, meaning that we are burning off fewer calories.

From the age of 30 years onward, the average weight gain is around a pound a year. That may not sound like much. But between the ages of 30 and 60 that's an extra 30 pounds of weight that we're all lugging around!

Don't Worry, There's Good News Too!

After reading that litany of bad news, I wouldn't blame you if you're not feeling too optimistic about your physical future. Well, let me provide you with some good news . . .

You can do something about it.

You may not be able to reverse all of the effects of aging, but you can most definitely do enough to reclaim the energy, vitality, strength and muscle mass that you thought were gone forever. The bottom line is that you can't stop the aging process, but you can most definitely slow it down.

The process by which you will be able to thrive into your 40s, 50s, 60s and beyond begins with a mental makeover. Rather than viewing each passing year as an excuse to do less, feel less and be less, take the opposite view. Consider the natural declines that occur with aging as a personal challenge. Make it your determination to, each day, be better than the day before. Rather than dreading your next birthday, welcome it. Embrace your age, determined to do whatever it takes to optimize your physical self.

In short, view the glass as half full rather than half empty!

WHAT FITNESS CAN DO FOR YOU

The key to thriving in your older years can be summed up in the word 'fitness'. However, fitness has come to be defined within narrow parameters in recent decades. In the next section, we will unpack what total fitness encompasses. For now, though, we can consider it to be the result of a lifestyle that prioritizes physical and mental well-being.

When you move beyond your 40th birthday, there are a number of lifestyle factors that should underpin your fitness lifestyle. Consider the following 7 factors and think about how you stack up in regard to them. Do you:

- Get regular (at least 6 monthly) medical checkups?
- Not smoke?
- Get regular exercise?
- Eat sensibly and in moderation?
- Strive to maintain a balanced weight?
- Know how to relax?

- Drink alcohol in moderation?

Even though I haven't gotten specific in terms of what regular exercise should look like or what constitutes healthy nutrition and balanced weight, I want you to give yourself a rating out of 7 as to how you stack up against this list. If you are doing each of these things, give yourself a point. If not, don't.

Take a moment to think about how you score.

If you identify an area where you need work, that's ok. When you begin to put into practice the 7 foundations of total fitness, you will find it a lot a lot easier to make that change. For now, it's enough to realize that the need exists and you have the desire to do something about it.

So, what benefits will you get from taking on a total fitness program?

The benefits of fitness start on the inside and radiate outwards. After your first workout, you will begin to feel better about yourself. The fact that you are taking your health in your own hands will give you a feeling of control that is missing in many people's lives. Too often, people act as if their body is a runaway car that's out of control and heading for a cliff. Exercise allows you to slam on the brakes, throw the vehicle into reverse and then head back onto the freeway of life.

When you take control of your physical future in this way, you develop self-confidence. You'll begin to walk a little taller and prouder. After an exercise session, you will have a feeling of accomplishment. At the same time, feel good endorphins will flush through your body, producing a natural high that will set you up for a great day.

Your fitness program will make you physically stronger. If you are new to resistance exercise, you should be able to improve your strength level by as much as 40 percent over a 12-month period. That will not only offset natural age-related strength decline, it will provide you with the power to accomplish the tasks that many people who age struggle with. At the same time, increased levels of physical strength add to the confidence that is the hallmark of a well-adjusted, healthy individual.

Along with your increased strength will come larger and tighter muscles. The changes that a few extra pounds of lean muscle tissue to a person's body composition makes can be quite dramatic. Adding some lean muscle to your shoulders, pectorals, back and quadriceps won't turn you into a bodybuilder but it will help you to sculpt the athletic type of physique that tells others that you care about your body and know how to look after it.

The more muscle you carry on your body, the less likely you will be to carry excess body fat. That's because muscle is very energy dependent. It takes about five times more energy to preserve an ounce of muscle than it does an ounce of fat. So, putting on muscle will speed up your metabolism, countering yet another of the natural effects of aging.

THE 7 FOUNDATIONS OF TOTAL FITNESS

The majority of people who work out put all of their energies into one particular form of fitness. For some it could be training with weights, while others spend the majority of their workout time in the cardio area or pounding the pavement as distance runners. However, the combination of decades of research and in the trenches experience has made it abundantly clear that the anti-aging benefits of fitness require a holistic approach to exercise.

A holistic approach means giving equal emphasis to each of the following 7 types of fitness:

1. Strength
2. Flexibility
3. Mobility
4. Stability
5. Agility
6. Endurance
7. Nutrition

These 7 foundations of total fitness can be considered a pension for your body and future function. The more you put into it, the more you get back!

Let's drill down on these foundations, one by one...

Strength

We haven't traditionally associated strength training with seniors. Yet, increasing the strength of the skeletal muscles has been shown to be profoundly beneficial as we age. In the past, the few seniors who discovered the benefits of strength training did so as part of their rehab program after an injury or accident. We now know that proactively beginning a strength training program in your 40s or 50s can help prevent those accidents or injuries from occurring in the first place.

Studies conducted over the past decade have shown that regular strength training can significantly reduce the symptoms of the following age - related conditions:

- Arthritis
- Poor balance
- Diabetes
- Osteoporosis
- Obesity
- Back pain
- Breathing problems
- Depression
- Dementia

In addition to making you far less likely to suffer from these and other health conditions, strength training will make you far more functional in your everyday tasks. A meta study out of the

Department of Occupational Therapy at Indiana University-Purdue University Indianapolis analyzed 121 trials involving 6,700 study participants between the ages of 60 and 80. The researchers concluded that seniors who participated in strength training workouts two to three times per week consistently outperformed those who didn't on common daily movements.

Strength training has been shown to improve emotional makeup and to promote better sleep. It also builds self-esteem and self-efficacy. Researchers are still trying to determine the reasons why strength training has such a positive powerful effect on the mind yet are unanimous that it is as effective as medication at relieving depression.

Flexibility

Flexibility is the ability of your muscles, ligaments and tendons to elongate to their maximum potential. Flexible muscles are stretchy and pliable.

If you don't have good flexibility, such everyday activities as getting out of bed, bending down to pick up a child or squatting down to lift a heavy object can become more demanding. A lack of adequate flexibility can also impair your athletic ability, as you will be unable to reach the full potential, strength and power of your muscles.

Flexibility Benefits

Increased Range of Motion: Range of motion is the distance and direction your joints can move. Consistent flexibility training will increase the range of motion of your joints and muscles. It does this by lengthening the muscles and opening the joints. As a result, you'll be able to stretch further in all directions while remaining pain free.

Decreased Risk of Injury: People with flexible muscles are less likely to become injured during physical activity.

Reduced Muscle Soreness: Flexibility training helps to reduce muscle soreness after you exercise. When you stretch after your workout, you keep your muscles loose and relaxed.

Mobility

Mobility is strength through the full range of motion of an exercise. Unlike flexibility, it relies on the muscle alone to produce the range of movement. So, a flexible person may be able to raise his straightened leg quite high with the assistance of their arm. A mobile person, however, will be able to manipulate their leg or other muscle without any help at all.

Many people who focus exclusively on strength training are strong through a limited range of a muscle's motion. Others are very mobile in parts of the body but not in others. We can think of cyclists with well-developed and mobile legs but poor development and mobility in the upper body.

Total fitness requires balanced mobility throughout the whole body.

Stability

By the time you reach the age of 40 you will very likely have developed a number of muscular imbalances throughout your body. This is the result of decades of doing the same actions over and over again. For many people, this is seen as a propensity to lean forward, hunch over and carry themselves with extremely poor posture. The result is muscular imbalance and instability.

When our body is unstable, some muscles are stronger and more flexible than others. We develop what are referred to as overactive and underactive muscles. The over reliance on our overactive muscles makes the imbalance worse every day. It not only robs us of our stability and balance but sets us up for injury.

Stability training focuses on how to stabilize the body and how to move correctly. It prepares a person to react with optimized reflexes to any situation while maintaining proper joint alignment.

Agility

Agility is the ability to move, not only freely and easily but also quickly and gracefully. Being agile means you can feel fitter and more vibrant than ever before! Agility training is vital for professional athletes to perform at a high level but also for everyday folk as well. Regular agility training will lead to enhanced speed and alertness.

There is no better form of exercise to enhance your balance and coordination than agility training. Agility exercises will also help you develop greater eye - hand and foot coordination and help prevent other injuries. As you will discover later in this book, agility training can also be a lot of fun!

Endurance

Muscular endurance relates to the body's ability to exert force over a period of time. It is the difference between being able to do a one repetition squat with a maximum weight and the ability to maintain the wall sit position for 10 minutes. The squat demonstrates the strength of your quadriceps while the wall sit reveals the endurance of that muscle.

Muscular endurance is closely linked to the concept of physical stamina - the ability to sustain an activity for a prolonged period. The more stamina you have, the greater your ability will be to carry out such everyday tasks as washing your car or raking up the leaves in your yard. You'll be able to continue an activity without feeling fatigued or exhausted. And when the grandkids come over, you will have the energy to get active with them without feeling like you need respirator relief after they've gone.

Muscular endurance training, in which you use a lighter load for higher repetitions, will increase the health of your bones and joints. The reduced likelihood of muscular fatigue will also lessen your likelihood of suffering a fatigue related injury or accident.

Cardiovascular endurance is another vital aspect of total fitness. It will help you to sustain aerobic exercise and is an indication of the health of your heart and lungs. The more cardiovascular endurance you have, the more efficiently your heart is able to pump oxygenated blood to your muscles.

Nutrition

Your body is made from the nutrients contained in food:

- Water
- Protein
- Carbohydrate
- Fat
- Vitamins
- Minerals

Nutrition is the science of how our bodies utilize food. It boils down to two things:

1. Food's ability to produce energy to allow us to function
2. The nutrients we need to build, maintain and repair the organs and systems in our bodies.

When you put 'unhealthy' foods into your mouth day after day, your body will eventually start to suffer. This can lead to numerous health issues that we will explore in chapter nine.

Everyone has their own idea of what constitutes good nutrition. We just need to look at the wide disparity among diet types to confirm this. They run the full spectrum from zero carbs to zero fat and back again. It's no wonder that so many people are so confused when it comes to just what to put into their mouths to promote health and fitness!

When thinking about your nutrition, it is helpful to understand the four important criteria that all good nutrition plans must meet. They must:

- Control energy balance
- Provide nutrient density
- Achieve healthy body composition
- Be outcome based

While other factors, such as exercise, sleep and lifestyle habits all affect our health and wellness, their effect is minimal in comparison to nutrition. That's why we all need to apply the four basic criteria of nutrition in order to provide our bodies with the fuel that it needs to operate optimally.

KEY POINTS

- As you age, your body naturally becomes less efficient. Changes you will go through include losing muscle mass, slowing of your metabolism, and producing less testosterone.
- You have the power, through exercise, to slow down the aging process.
- Exercise will improve your self - image and your self-confidence.
- Regular exercise will make you physically and mentally stronger, improve your bone strength, body composition, coordination and balance.
- Exercise will boost the efficiency of your heart and lungs and make you far less likely to succumb to age-related disease.
- The 7 foundations of total fitness are strength, mobility, flexibility, stability, agility, endurance and nutrition.

2

DEVELOPING A MINDSET FOR SUCCESS

E very action you take begins with a thought. When it comes to making changes to your physical health, the way you think about yourself and about the world at large is critical to your success or failure. Unless you get your mind primed for success, you will fail to achieve your goals, regardless of what else you do.

We are living in an out of control world. People are so busy nowadays that they hardly have time to think - let alone breathe - before they're off to the next appointment, the next pick up or the next thing on their to do list. As a result, many people accept what happens to them as inevitable, as something over which they have little control, or as pure chance. They pile on weight, fail to stick to an exercise program or ditch their clean eating plan when the pressure comes on like waves that are

TOTAL FITNESS AFTER 40 | 35

being tossed about in an ocean of ill-disciplined self-indulgence and mediocrity.

The truth is very different. Every person - me and you included - has the power to take control of their destiny. We are not controlled by circumstance, unless we choose to be. This is especially so when it comes to the most personal and precious thing we possess - our health.

A balanced life, one in which we are giving proper attention to maintaining our physical, emotional, spiritual and psychological health, is within the grasp of each one of us. All we need is the courage to reach out and grasp hold of it.

Often the roots of people's inability to find success is rooted in negative self-talk. We are talking to ourselves all day long - you're probably doing it as you read these words. In fact, on the average day, you think some 60,000 thoughts. The majority of them are repetitive. Now for the startling part – most people's inner talk is predominantly negative. As a result, they are constantly feeding themselves with pessimism. They tell themselves 'I'll always be fat', 'It'll never work for me because I love food too much', or 'I can't do that'.

Learning to reprogram our minds to eliminate negativity is fundamental to taking control of our physical destiny. Spend the time to do that and everything else - the physical things like exercising and eating - will be so deeply ingrained in your psyche that you will be programmed for success. A lean, supple, energetic body will soon follow.

To think about . . .

What is the state of your inner self talk? Over the next 24 hours, consciously track your inner dialogue to gauge how many thoughts are couched in negativity. Whenever you catch one, kick it out and replace it with a positive affirmation.

Here are four more strategies to overcome negative self-talk:

- Question your thinking; before condemning yourself when you slip up, pause and question your thinking. If it's irrational, dismiss it!
- Eliminate self-prejudice; self-prejudice causes us to distort reality. To counter it, try to judge yourself as if you were an impartial observer.
- Own your imperfections; stop expecting perfection from yourself. Accept your faults and move on.
- Build your self-esteem; engage in new and different activities, such as playing sports and exercising.

THE POWER OF VISUALIZATION

A major key to achieving success is the ability to plant in the forefront of your mind vivid imagery of yourself successfully doing the thing that you want to achieve. A few years ago, mental imagery, also known as visualization, was the domain of professional athletes and self-help gurus. In recent times, however, there has been an increasing appreciation for the positive effects of mental imagery on goal attainment among the everyday exerciser.

When you regularly visualize yourself accomplishing your goals in your 'mind's eye', you provide a powerful stimulus to success. All you need to do is to utilize your imagination and focus to mentally rehearse the attainment of your goals. Start at the daily level and do it while you are lying in bed before you get up in the morning. See yourself doing everything that you need to in order to have a perfect goal attainment day, from springing out of bed, enjoying a healthy nutritious breakfast, powering through an invigorating, calorie depleting work-out and then enjoying an energy restoring post workout shake.

When you're lying in bed at night, you should undertake another mental imagery session. See yourself having accomplished your end goal with the body, the strength and the energy that you are working towards. Create a crystal-clear image of this new you and embrace the feelings that go with it – the self-confidence, the energy and the joy of accomplishment.

SMART GOAL SETTING

Most of us aren't very good at setting goals. Fortunately, an excellent template has been devised to help us get it right. It is summed up in the acronym SMART, which stands for:

- Specific
- Measurable
- Achievable
- Realistic
- Time Bound

Let's consider them one by one . . .

Specific

Your goals need to be specifically defined. If your goal is generalized, it will be impossible to know when you have achieved it. That is why your goal needs to have an element of detail. So, rather than setting the goal that you want to 'get fit', drill down to a specific goal like 'running a half marathon'.

Note, too, that it is always best to couch your goal in concrete, definite rather than hopeful terminology. So, rather than saying "My goal is to run a half marathon", rephrase it as "I will run a half marathon."

Measurable

As well as being specific, your goals also need to be quantifiable. That is why losing weight is not a goal. Unless you quantify the amount of weight you want to lose, you will never know when you get there. So, here again, you need to drill down. State how much weight you are going to lose or, even better, what body fat percentage you are going to achieve. That way you will be able to monitor your progress and know if you are on track to the goal's achievement.

Achievable

It's great to aim for the stars, but aiming for another galaxy is to merely set yourself up for failure. There is a definite link between achievable goals, realistic timelines and stepping stone goals. In this regard, there is no better example than Arnold Schwarzenegger.

As a teenager living in Thal, Austria, Arnold set goals that everyone who he told them to thought were ridiculous; to become the best built man in the world and then become a famous Hollywood movie star. Even the idea of getting to America was as distant as traveling to the moon for rural Austrians in the 1950s. Yet, Arnold had the ability to break down his major long-term goals into smaller goals, each of which fed into the next goal. In fact, he was able to break down his goals to such an extent that his daily actions, everything he ate and every rep he performed in the gym, were connected with the fulfillment of his major goal. That fueled his desire to steadily work toward the fulfillment of goals that, on their face, appeared to be unachievable.

Realistic

A realistic goal is one that you are actually able to achieve. If you are in your forties, your goal to become a fighter pilot is probably not going to happen. Instead, modify your goal to something that is more realistic, like learning to become a pilot and flying a private plane. If you are a natural weight trainer, and you're not six foot five, you are not going to end up with 24-inch biceps, no matter how many sets of curls you do! But you will be able to develop an extremely impressive set of guns in the mid to late teens.

Time Bound

We've already touched upon the importance of time in relation to your goals in terms of keeping the goal achievable. So, while you shouldn't set yourself up for failure by having an unrealistic timeline, it is vital that you do have some sort of time element to your goal. Without a time-frame, you do not have a goal at all, only a vague ambition. But with one, you have a deadline. As a result, your sense of urgency increases and you are more likely to attain your goal.

Write your goal like this . . .

It is 1st May and I have just completed a half marathon

Writing your goal in the first-person present tense is very powerful. By re-reading that goal several times daily you will be transmitting the message to your subconscious, where it will go to work to fuel your drive to succeed!

LEARNING TO LOVE EXERCISE

Most people view exercise as a means to an end. Most of them don't enjoy the experience. To them, exercise is like bad tasting medicine that they must take in order to protect their health. The sooner they get it over with, the better. If you have that viewpoint, you will never succeed in achieving your fitness goals.

Here are four keys to learning to love exercise.

Forget the Past

Over 70% of Americans are either sedentary or not receiving the minimum amount of recommended exercise. Despite knowing that they should be working out, a lot of these people simply don't like exercise. This attitude is typically formed very early on in life.

By putting aside the bad experiences you have had in the past and focusing on new things that you find enjoyable, you'll be able to make your mind over. The key is to find an activity that you really enjoy doing and use it as the foundation for your exercise session.

Pace Yourself

When you first start working out, don't go full out straight away. If you exhaust yourself straight off the bat, you'll be adding fuel to the idea that you don't like exercising. Take it steady and build up gradually, enjoying the training along the way.

Exercise is movement. It's not confined to the gym or a set block of workout time. It could be walking, swimming, playing basketball or any other activity that you enjoy that will get your heart rate up for 30 minutes.

Ditch the Excuses

A lot of people tell themselves that they don't have time for exercise. We're all incredibly busy with more and more demands coming in on us all the time. But exercise needs to be a priority in your schedule. It is, after all, the key to everything else. Unless your body is maintained you will not be able to do all of those other things that are tugging at your time. For that reason you must schedule your workout into your calendar as non-negotiable 'you' time. Let people know that you are not available during those times.

Sometimes we have excellent intentions to exercise, but simply can't build up the motivation. The key, again, is to find something that you enjoy doing. If you enjoy it, motivation will not be a problem. A great way to overcome lack of motivation is to ask a friend to be your workout buddy. If you know that someone is waiting for you, you're much more likely to turn up at the exercise venue than if you're just relying on your own motivation level to get you there.

A trap that people often fall into is to put barriers in front of their ability to exercise. They do this by telling themselves that they must buy something before they can begin. It could be new shoes, gym clothes or a stopwatch that they have told themselves they need before they can start training. These are really just ways to procrastinate.

The reality is that you don't need any special equipment in order to get started on an exercise routine. Put the excuses aside, save your money, and just get started.

Overcome Insecurities

A lot of people feel very self-conscious when it comes to exercise. They can easily let their own personal insecurities hold them back. They'll convince themselves that others will laugh at them. That is almost certainly not going to be the case. If you've felt these insecurities, you simply have to put aside what you think other people might be thinking and just go ahead and do the things that you've always wanted to do.

BUILDING THE EXERCISE HABIT

It's been said that habits are like a warm bath on a cold night – easy to get into, and hard to get out of. While that may be true of bad habits, many people find it extremely difficult to get started with good habits – and then to stick with them. However, by breaking down the latest research on habit formation we can identify a simple three step process which will allow anyone to cultivate new habits.

Researchers at the Massachusetts Institute of Technology have done a lot of research on habits. They have broken down the process of habit formation into three key steps which they call the habit loop. These three parts are . . .

1. Cue, which is the trigger that starts the habit
2. Routine, which is the habit itself
3. Reward, which is the benefit you get from doing the habit

Habits will not be formed without cues. This is true of both good and bad habits. So, we need to work hard to trigger the right sort of cues – those that will lead to our good habits and not our bad habits. When it comes to cues there are four main types – location, time, the actions of others and the action that you took immediately prior to starting the habit. Let's take a quick look at each of them.

Location is a major habit driver. Many habits are nothing more than responses to our environment. You can manipulate your environment to help develop your new habit. Let's say your desired new habit is to start going to the gym in the morning before work. Your key environment is your bedroom. Set it up to make it easy to get out the door rather than staying in bed. Lay out your gym clothes, have your trainers out and ready to slip on and place your gym bag by the front door.

Time cues are very common. We become conditioned to automatically do things at certain times of the day. We can use this to our advantage to trigger new habits. Tie your new habit to a time and day. Let's say that your new habit is to go to the gym three mornings a week before work. So, if it's Monday at 6:00 am, that triggers you to get up and get moving. It doesn't matter how you're feeling or what you'd rather do, it's automatic!

The actions of others are powerful influences on our habits. But recent research has shown just how pervasive that influence is. One study, published in the New England Journal of Medicine, revealed that people who have an obese friend are 57 percent more likely to become obese themselves. So, it is vital that you surround yourself with people who will support your habit. With our morning gym habit, it is a great idea to find a workout buddy, and to have people at work and home who ask about how your workouts are going and give you encouragement to keep it up. Getting a text from your friend at 6:10 in the morning to wish you well on your workout is a powerful incentive to make it happen.

The action you take immediately prior to the habit action is very important. The experts call this habit stacking. This is when you pair a desired new habit with another one which you have already mastered. Let's go back to the early morning gym habit. You may have already developed the habit of having a coffee first thing in the morning. Pair this with grabbing your workout bag. Write this down as an affirmation this way . . .

As soon as I've had my morning coffee, I'll grab my workout bag and leave the house.

Notice that the action cue is very specific. 'As soon as' leaves no room for wishy washiness.

The second phase of the habit loop is the actual performance of the habit. To help make it stick you should do it the same way and with the same rituals every time. We all have little rituals we perform before we do things. In the gym example, it could be the way that you set yourself before doing a squat, or the number of breaths you take before you lift the bar off the rack. You should also perform your habit in the same place every time.

The third and final phase of the habit loop is the reward. This is based on the scientific principle of operant conditioning. This states that if you get a good feeling after you do a habit, you will continue to do it. The types of rewards that we give to ourselves are individual. Just provide yourself with a small celebration every time you perform your habit. This could be as simple as crossing off your gym visits on a calendar over a period of a week, or month. Then, at the end of that time period you might purchase that book you've been wanting or go out for a restaurant meal. You don't have to continue to reward yourself extrinsically forever. Once the habit is established, your rewards will become intrinsic. For example, going back to our workout example, the endorphin rush, self-esteem and bodily improvements that you experience will be rewards in themselves.

Developing a new habit, it has been often said, takes 21 days. Yet, there is no science behind that number. For some it will become habitual sooner than that, for others it will take more time. Rather than focusing on a number, like 21 days, just focus on repeating the habit loop until you don't even have to think about it.

So, how do you stick to a new habit? The first way is to develop new habits one at a time. Make a list of all of the new habits you want to develop, then prioritize them. Start with the most important and focus exclusively on implementing that habit before moving to the next one. Another important tip is to break your habit down into mini-habits. With the gym example, we've already identified some key mini habits – setting out your gym clothes and getting your bag ready the night before, mixing up your pre-workout drink, doing your warm-up. Focus on doing those things and the rest will follow.

Creating the Ideal Workout Program

Now that you know how to cement in your new exercise habit, let's talk about creating the ideal program in order to maximize your workout time while ensuring proper recovery and covering all areas of fitness.

The FITT Principle helps us to achieve those goals. FITT stands for:

- Frequency
- Intensity
- Time
- Type

Frequency

The starting point to constructing your workout program is deciding how often you will exercise. The current general recommendations for physical activity are 150 minutes of aerobic activity week at moderate-intensity exercise. That equates to about half an hour a day, five days a week. That activity should include doing a range of physical activities that incorporate fitness, strength, balance and flexibility. However, such activities as gardening and playing sport should also be included in your total exercise count. Including these types of activities will help to make sure that you are getting the proper balance between exercise and recovery.

Alternatively, it is recommended that you do 75 minutes of vigorous intensity exercise on a weekly basis. On top of that, you should do muscle strengthening activity on at least two days per week.

Intensity

Intensity relates to how hard your workout is. Your intensity level depends on the type of exercise you are doing and your training goal. Intensity depends on your current fitness level and your skill level. You can adjust the intensity level of your workout by:

- Changing the resistance amount
- Adjusting the number of sets and repetitions
- Varying the cadence of movement
- Changing the rest time between sets and exercises
- Performing intensity enhancing techniques such as supersets, drop sets and pre-exhaustion training

Time

Time relates to the amount of time that you are investing into your training sessions. When it comes to cardiovascular exercise, the general guidelines recommend doing between 20 and 60 minutes. However, this will depend on the intensity of the exercise you are doing. Steady state low intensity cardio, such as walking on a treadmill, can be done for up to an hour at a time. In contrast, high intensity interval training (HIIT), which involves short sprints followed by even shorter rest intervals, should only last for a maximum of 20 minutes.

Varying the length and intensity of your cardio workouts will promote total fitness.

Strength training workouts will usually last between 30 and 60 minutes, depending on whether you are training designated body parts or your whole body.

Type

There are many different types of exercise that you can do to work the various elements that comprise total fitness. However, all of them can be divided into two broad categories

- Aerobic
- Anaerobic

Aerobic

Aerobic exercise primarily benefits the cardiovascular system. It strengthens the heart and lungs while, at the same time, burning off excess calories. Examples of aerobic exercise are walking, cycling and skipping.

The word aerobic means 'with oxygen'. When you perform aerobic exercise, your muscles are getting enough oxygen to produce the required energy. This type of exercise is done at a steady, moderate pace and can be sustained for a long period of time.

Aerobic exercise primarily uses slow twitch muscle fibers and is best for cardiovascular health and endurance training.

Anaerobic

Anaerobic exercise is high intensity, short duration exercise that you cannot keep up for a long time. Weight lifting and sprinting are examples of anaerobic exercise. The word anaerobic means 'without oxygen.' With this type of exercise, the oxygen demands on your muscles are greater than the oxygen supply. This results in the production of lactate and the stopping of the exercise.

Anaerobic exercise is best to work your musculoskeletal system.

The FITT Principle will help you to continue training at optimal effectiveness over time. You should begin your exercise habit with a light frequency, low intensity workout, relatively short time per session and two types of exercise (one aerobic and the other anaerobic). An example would be to walk three times per week for 30 minutes each time and to accompany this with two full body strength training sessions.

As your body adapts to your training, you need to adjust your workouts in order to place increasing demands on your body. If you keep doing the same things, month in and month out, your body will have no reason to respond by getting fitter and stronger. When you decide that you need to adjust your workout, you should change one or more of the elements of FITT. For example, you could:

- Increase the frequency of walking to 5 days; or
- Increase the intensity by speed walking; or
- Increase the time by walking for 45 minutes per session; or
- Changing the exercise type by cycling.

To be safe, you should only change one thing at a time. Once you have done a week or so of the adjusted workout, you can change another aspect to progress your fitness.

ENERGY SYSTEMS

Every breath you take, every move you make and every thought you think requires energy. When you work out, it needs it more than when you are at rest. All of the energy that allows you to function comes from the food that you eat. That food is broken down in the body to produce energy in the form of ATP (adenosine triphosphate).

ATP is stored in our muscle cells, but only in very limited amounts. That stored ATP will only supply the energy you need to exercise for a matter of seconds. To continue to function, the cells then require more ATP being made by the body.

There are three systems that the body can use to produce ATP:

- The ATP-PCR system
- The glycolytic system
- The oxidative system

The ATP-PCR and the glycolytic system are both anaerobic because they do not require oxygen. The oxidative system does require oxygen to make ATP.

The ATP-PCR system allows for exercise between 5-15 seconds. The ATP stored in the muscle will power up to the first five seconds. The salt phosphate (PCR) attaches to ATP to provide another 10 seconds or so of energy.

Once the ATP-PCR system is used up, the body switches to the glycolytic system. Now the body relies upon glycogen, which is the broken-down form of carbohydrate, to make ATP. This is achieved through the process of glycolysis. During glycolysis, lactate is produced, along with hydrogen ions. These are responsible for the muscle burn and fatigue you feel when sprinting or lifting heavy weights.

The glycolytic system will sustain you for up to two minutes of exercise. After that, the body switches to the oxidative system. With this system, ATP is produced using two mechanisms:

- The Krebs cycle
- The electron transport chain

The oxidative system produces ATP more slowly than the other two systems, but it will provide energy for a greater duration. This explains why you can run slowly for a long period of time, but sprint for only a short period of time, before you are exhausted.

It is possible to exercise each of the energy systems to be more efficient. Doing explosive plyometric moves like box jumps will improve your ATP-PCR system. Circuit training, where you move from one exercise to the next with little to no rest, will make your glycolytic system more efficient, and performing 20-30 minute cardio sessions of moderate intensity, such as walking, jogging or biking, can improve your oxidative system.

THE IMPORTANCE OF YOUR TRAINING HEART RATE

Zone heart rate training is based on exercise intensity and heart rate zones. There are five heart rate zones that are each based upon a person's maximum heart rate. While it is impossible to precisely work out your maximum heart rate, there are a number of formulas to provide you with a close estimate. The most common formula for working out your maximum heart rate is to subtract your heart rate from 220.

So, if you are 40 years of age, your max heart rate is . . .

$$220 - 40 = 180$$

Here's an overview of the 5 heart rate training zones . . .

Zone One

The first training heart rate zone represents a light intensity of training, such as going for an evening walk. This training heart rate zone is 50-60% of your max heart rate.

For our 40 year old exerciser, Zone One would be between 90 and 108 beats per minute.

Zone Two

The second training zone represents a medium intensity level, such as jogging or rollerblading. This training heart rate is 60-70% of your max heart rate.

For our 40 year old exerciser, Zone Two would be between 108 and 126 beats per minute.

Zone Three

The third training zone represents a light to medium intensity level, such as power walking and cycling. This training heart rate is 70-80% of your max heart rate.

For our 40 year old exerciser, Zone Three would be between 126 and 144 beats per minute.

Zone Four

The fourth training zone represents a high intensity level, such as sprinting and uphill cycling. This training heart rate is 80-90% of your max heart rate.

For our 40 year old exerciser, Zone Four would be between 144 and 162 beats per minute.

Beginner exercisers should not train in Zone 4 until they have built up their aerobic fitness level with around six months of training.

Zone Five

The fifth training zone represents your maximum heart rate. This is where your heart, lungs and respiratory functioning are all operating at full capacity. Only athletes who are at an extremely high level of fitness should train at their maximum heart rate. Examples of training at Zone 5 include Tabata style High Intensity Interval Training (HIIT). Zone 5 represents 90-100% of your maximum heart rate. For our 40 year old exerciser, Zone 5 would be between 162 and 180 beats per minute.

Keep in mind that the calculation for your max heart rate is just an estimate, so there is some margin of error. Over time, as you train more, your exercise intensity may have to change for each of the zones. For example, beginner exercisers who go for a light jog may be in Zone 3. But, as they continue to work out, their body will adapt and their fitness improves, so that in three to five weeks that same jog will only put them in Zone 2. That means that you have significantly improved your aerobic fitness level. Using a heart rate monitor is an easy way to track the heart rate zone you are working in, and your improvements in aerobic fitness over time.

KEY POINTS

- You have the power to be the master of your physical destiny
- Eliminate negative self-talk
- Use visualization to enforce your positive mindset
- Create SMART goals that are specific, measurable, achievable, realistic and time bound
- Learn to love exercise by forgetting the past, pacing yourself, ditching excuses and overcoming insecurities
- Build the exercise habit with cues, routines and rewards
- Use the FITT Principle to create your ideal workout program
- Work through all three energy systems to achieve total fitness
- Vary your training heart rate zone for total cardiovascular fitness

3

STRENGTH - YOU ARE STRONGER THAN YOU KNOW!

I'd like to begin this chapter with a bold declarative statement . . .

No matter your age or ability now, you NEED to take up strength training and perform it consistently over the course of the rest of your life. It is never too late to start and, as soon as you do, your body and your mind will start to reap immediate benefits.

Now, let's find out why I can make such an unequivocal recommendation.

When we consider aging and the diseases of modern civilization, we find that almost all of them are related to muscle loss that occurs with aging, or sarcopenia. It has also been shown that reversal or improvement in these diseases is preceded by the reclaiming of muscle mass and strength. As a result, for some reason that is still not fully understood, muscle and strength seem to be the key to maintaining our health as we age.

The American Council of Aging have identified the following 10 biomarkers of health:

1. Muscle Mass
2. Strength
3. Bone Density
4. Bone Composition
5. Blood Lipids
6. Hemodynamics
7. Glucose Control
8. Aerobic Capacity
9. Gene Expression
10. Brain Factors

How many of those essential biomarkers of health do you think strength training benefits?

Even if regular strength training improved 2 or 3 of these areas, wouldn't you agree that it would be a worthwhile activity to engage in?

Well, the fact is that strength training will produce marked improvement in ALL of these areas. That is not only remarkable, but also unequalled by any other activity. And that is why strength training needs to form the foundation of your health and wellness lifestyle.

Let's drill down on each of these essential health biomarkers to see just how strength training can help.

Muscle Mass / Strength

As people get older, they become more likely to fall and lose their balance. In fact, in 2016, falls became the number one cause of traumatic death in people over the age of 65. The common perception is that the elderly are more prone to falling due to arthritis and stiffness. But that is not the case. It is actually related to the loss of muscle, and in particular a type of muscle called Type II fiber. This type of muscle fiber is capable of producing a lot of force suddenly. Yet, these fibers are the most prone to atrophy and strength loss when they are not used.

When your Type II fibers are strong and numerous, they act rapidly and strongly as a counter when you lean forward or go off balance in order to right your balance and prevent a fall. This happens without your conscious awareness. But when you lose the functionality of these Type II fibers, that counter doesn't kick in and you fall over.

Skeletal muscle is the largest and most active endocrine / immunogenic organ in the human body. Your muscles are constantly sending chemical signals out to all of the tissues of your body. Those signals are vital to the optimal functioning of those tissues. As a result, strength training has benefits far beyond those related specifically to muscle mass and strength.

So, how beneficial is strength training to the restoration of muscle mass and strength?

In one study, a 30 percent loss of strength that had accumulated over 12 years was restored with just one year of strength training. As incredible as that turnaround sounds, it is, in fact, a modest result! Most people, when they follow an optimized strength training program will actually be able to improve their strength levels by as much as 300 percent in a 12-month period.

Bone Density

It has been known for some time that strength training can dramatically improve bone density. It used to be thought that this was due to increased mechanical load and stress on the bone with this type of exercise, but now researchers have discovered that it is in fact due to myokine signaling. When they are being stressed through exercise, muscles send out a hormonal signal to bones that promotes increased strength. The good news is that this signaling is not proportionate to the load that is on the muscle, which means that you don't have to overload the muscle with very heavy weights to promote bone density improvement.

Body Composition

Our body tissues are in competition with each other for nutrients. Myokines that are released from skeletal muscle as a result of strength training stress force the body to prioritize lean muscle tissue in nutrient allocation. The nutrients available will flow toward preserving the muscle rather than body fat. Strength training induced myokine increase also enhances fatty acid uptake from your fat cells as well as promoting an increase in glucose uptake and a speeding up of your metabolism. It has also been shown to activate insulin signaling. This mimics the action of the hormone leptin, decreasing inflammation in your body.

Strength training has also been shown to increase the release of the myokine Interleukin 15 from muscle cells. This myokine signals your existing fat cells and triggers a chemical called uncoupling protein to convert white fat (which is essentially an energy storing depot and precursor of inflammation) into brown fat, which speeds up the action of the mitochondria in the cell to produce more energy and, therefore, burn off more fat.

Blood Lipids

When it comes to blood lipids, doctors typically measure total cholesterol, HDL (good) and LDL (bad) cholesterol. Strength training will raise your HDL and lower your LDL cholesterol levels. More importantly, though, it opposes inflammatory myokines and controls insulin sensitivity and serum insulin levels. This is a major preventative against cardiovascular disease, which, according to the Center for Disease Control and Prevention, is the leading cause of death in the USA today.

Hemodynamics

Hemodynamics is all to do with blood flow. This is an area where strength training really outshines aerobic or steady state exercise. Starling's Law of the Heart describes how the heart functions; our heart works in a similar way to our septic system. It works optimally if the volume on the input side equals the volume on the output side. So, the cardiac output out of the left side of your heart is directly proportional to the amount of blood that is delivered to the right side of the heart. In other words, if 500ml of blood comes in, then 500ml will go out.

Coronary arteries come off the base of aorta and supply blood flow to the heart. The blood that returns to your heart through the coronary arteries is very passive. All the blood below the level of your heart gets there through muscle contraction and a one-way valve network that pushes the blood back to the heart. The intense muscular contraction involved in strength training enhances venous blood flow to the right side of the heart, which increases the blood volume that is pumped in the heart. In harmony with Starling's Law, this also increases the volume of blood that is pumped out of the left side of the heart. This also has the benefit of enhancing the backwash, which floods the coronary arteries and determines coronary artery blood flow.

Furthermore, the stronger the muscles, the more intense the muscle contractions that shunt blood up to the heart and the greater the amount of blood that will be pumped around the body will be. Strength training also decreases blood pressure.

In these ways, strength training has proven to be hugely beneficial for people with coronary artery disease.

Blood Glucose Control

Skeletal muscle is the biggest glucose reservoir in the body. When you do high intensity strength training, you exhaust your muscle's glycogen stores. This demands improved insulin sensitivity and improved glucose transport into the working muscle cell. This is the opposite to the metabolic syndrome that happens when we eat a bad diet and become sedentary.

Aerobic Capacity

Aerobic metabolism happens in the mitochondria of our cells. But aerobic metabolism cannot happen without anaerobic metabolism delivering its substrate, pyruvate, to the cell. Yet anaerobic metabolism delivers pyruvate to the cell at a rate faster than aerobic metabolism can handle it. So, the only way to maximally improve aerobic capacity is by doing hard anaerobic exercise such as - you guessed it! - strength training, that delivers pyruvate as fast as it can be aerobically metabolized.

Gene Expression

A landmark study in 2007 led by Dr. Simon Melov of the University of Southern California found that resistance training reduces aging in skeletal muscle tissue. The researchers identified 176 genes related to aging that reverted back to youthful levels of expression after just 26 weeks of strength training.

This was the first scientific study to show that it is possible to reverse aging at the genetic level.

How?

With strength training!

Brain Factors

Brain derived neurotrophic factor (BDNF) is a myokine that is known as the memory myokine. BDNF is low in people with Alzheimer's, depression and obesity, and is an independent marker for morbidity. Strength training has been shown to increase BDNF levels. Scientists do not know just how the mechanism works, but it is clear that BDNF produced in skeletal muscles is able to cross the blood brain barrier and produce significant cognitive benefits.

What is Strength Training?

We've seen that strength training addresses all ten of the biomarkers of health. That makes it unequalled in its ability to produce health benefits, especially as we age. So, now that we know that strength training is something that you should be doing, let's take a look at just what strength training involves.

Strength can be thought of like an iceberg. The part of the iceberg that is above the water is like the external strength that is seen when a person performs heavy lifts like the bench press or a deadlift. But hiding under the water, the 90 percent of your strength that is not outwardly visible has to do with the functional strength of the person's muscles as they work together. Often people who are very strong in one area, such as pressing overhead, have developed weaknesses in other areas, such as the glutes, hamstrings or lower back. As a result, they leave themselves open to imbalance injuries. They are also more likely to develop abnormal patterns of movement that sees them favoring their stronger muscles. This is often seen with poor posture which can result in problems like lower back pain.

The strength that is developed in your muscles is underpinned by the other 6 foundations of total fitness:

- Flexibility
- Mobility
- Stability
- Agility
- Endurance
- Nutrition

Strength training involves lifting and lowering weight in a controlled manner. You begin with a slow, gradual upload of resistance and then you work to make progressive resistance as you continue onward. You need to be lifting slowly and smoothly with the intent of using the resistance to bring about a deep level of fatigue in the working muscle.

When you place a strength training demand on the body, you are asking the body to make an adaptation to become stronger and more muscular in order to meet the demand in future. In this way, strength training is a stimulus. The adaptation that it stimulates requires time, recuperation and nutrients.

THE STRENGTH TRAINING PYRAMID

The Strength Training Pyramid is a graphic representation of the factors that should go into a properly structured exercise program. Here's what the pyramid looks like...

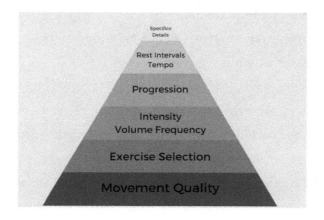

Let's consider the six levels of the Strength Pyramid one by one. At the bottom of the pyramid, we have Movement Quality.

MOVEMENT QUALITY

There are a number of different forms of exercise that you could do to improve your health. However, you only have a limited amount of time and energy to contribute to this part of your life. As a result, you need to select the form of movement that will give you the best bang for your buck - in other words, the quality of your exercise matters! For the reasons already presented in this chapter, if you had to produce just one form of exercise, that should be strength training.

But what sort of strength training should you do?

There are a number of options:

- Bodyweight training
- Resistance band training
- Dynamic tension free weight / machine training
- Isometric training

In terms of achieving the best biomechanical and anatomical benefits, the best form of strength training and the focus of this chapter is dynamic tension free weight and machine training. That is because dynamic tension strength training allows you to move a muscle through its complete biomechanical range of motion. As a result, the muscle lengthens and shortens to create muscle contraction following the natural strength curve of the muscle, which is hardest at the beginning of the exercise and easiest at the end of the exercise. You can also adjust free weights and resistance machines to a weight that is safe and suited to your strength on any given day.

In contrast, resistance band training reverses the natural strength curve, being easiest at the beginning and hardest at the end of the movement. If you do not have access to a gym or are going on holiday or a business trip, resistance bands are still a good alternative as they are small and easy to fit into a suitcase.

Isometric exercise does not move a muscle through its range of motion and instead involves static holds. This doesn't mean to say that they do not have significant benefits. They are still important for strength, muscle endurance, stability and involve the muscles to be constantly engaged during the exercise.

Bodyweight training is still very beneficial as it helps to improve strength, endurance, flexibility, balance and mobility. The problem with bodyweight training is that a lot of people simply do not have the strength to lift their own body weight. This can lead to very bad form and a high chance of injuries. For example: Sinking your pelvis during a press up due to a weak core can lead to lower back problems. A really handy piece of equipment to acquire is a suspension trainer. This can be used to aid bodyweight training exercises by controlling how much bodyweight resistance you use. Although not the focus of strength training in this book, I would highly recommend further looking into a suspension trainer.

NEXT UP IN THE PYRAMID IS EXERCISE SELECTION.

EXERCISE SELECTION

Correct selection of the exercises that you perform as part of your workout is critical in order to ensure that you are getting the maximum benefit from your training investment without causing injury to your body. Unfortunately, many of the exercises that are accepted as 'fundamental' to strength training do neither of those things. So, rather than simply doing what everyone else in the gym is doing, we need to approach the subject from an objective, scientific point of view.

There are a number of principles we can use based on biomechanical physics to rate how good an exercise is in terms of strength development and muscle stimulation. Here are 3 of them:

1. The exercise should allow the operating lever of the target muscle to move directly toward the origin of the muscle fiber. For example, the operating lever of a dumbbell curl is the forearm, and it moves toward the origin of the biceps which is the scapula.

2. The exercise should provide alignment between the direction of the resistance, the direction of the motion and the origin and insertion points of the muscle fiber. If we think about the latissimus dorsi muscle, the muscle fibers are mostly diagonal from their origin on the spine and their insertion on the upper inner part of the humerus (upper arm bone). Muscles always pull toward their origin, so the ideal movement for the lats is diagonally down from an angle where the arm is pulling at about 30 degrees down and in toward the hip. This is achieved with the One Arm Lat Pull In, rather than the Lat Pulldown, Chin Up or Seated Row, which are much more commonly seen in the gym, but none of which follow the direction of the muscle fibers.

Lat Pull In

1. The exercise should allow a muscle to move through its full range of motion. Let's consider the example of the deltoid (shoulder) muscles. There are three deltoid heads. The anterior (front) deltoid pulls the upper arm forward and upward. So its range of motion is from an arm position behind the torso and through to full arm extension in front of the body. The lateral (side) delts move the arms out to the side, while the posterior (rear) delt moves down and back. None of these ranges of

motions look anything like what you are doing when you perform the overhead press, which has traditionally been the 'go-to' exercise for the deltoids. The smart exerciser will choose exercises that follow the range of motion of the muscle in its natural movement.

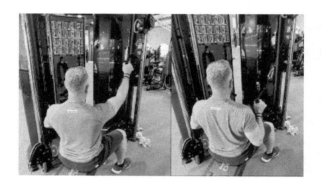

For the deltoids, those exercises are the following:

Cable Front Deltoid Press

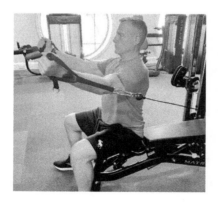

Rear Delt Cable Extension

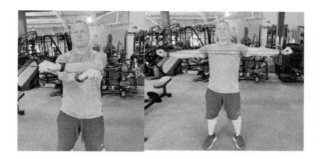

Cable Side Lateral Raise

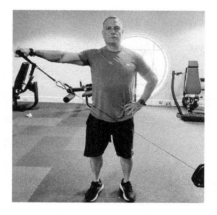

A lot of the exercises recommended later in this section have been selected because they follow these principles. Here are some examples of exercises that, although very common, do not align with the ideal principles outlined above. This compromises them in various ways. I'm not saying that you should never do these exercises, simply that there are more biomechanically beneficial options that come with a much reduced risk of injury as we age:

- Upright Rowing
- Preacher Barbell Curls
- Overhead Shoulder Press
- Barbell Squats
- Bent Over Barbell Row
- Barbell deadlifts
- Hanging Leg Raises

One reason the barbell deadlift can be so dangerous is that due to the bar being in front of your body, it forces your shoulders to protract forward, rounding the top of your spine. This also puts added load on your lower back. For an alternative, you can use what's known as a Hex or Trap bar. Your hands will now be at your sides which retracts the shoulders and engages your upper back more to take some of that load off the lower back. This will also engage the quadriceps more, but it's still a far safer option.

The next level in our strength training pyramid shows the importance of Intensity, Volume and Frequency.

INTENSITY, VOLUME, FREQUENCY

When you perform strength training exercises, you impose stress on the muscle. It is the adaptation to that stress that produces beneficial results. The reason that these adaptations occur is to prepare the muscle to meet that same stress level in future and be able to handle it. Unless your level of intensity is progressive, then you will not see a continual progression of benefits. That is because your body will already have adapted to the stress level.

Increasing the intensity of your workout can be achieved by increasing the resistance, increasing the time under tension (i.e. the amount of time you are contracting the muscle) or reducing the rest time between sets.

The volume of a strength training session relates to the total amount of work that you perform within a workout. It is possible to overtrain a muscle by doing too much just as it is possible to undertrain it by doing too little. The ideal volume for a muscle to elicit the maximum muscle building result seems to be 8-10 sets, with a rep range of between 6 and 20 reps. This wide rep range will allow you to stimulate all muscle fiber types, including Type II fiber, which we have already identified as being crucial in preventing falls and balance issues. You can also increase the volume of work by increasing your time under tension by taking longer to perform the movement, or adding isometric holds into each rep.

When designing our strength training program to achieve the correct intensity, volume and frequency, we need to consider metabolic stress. This describes the point when our muscles begin to fatigue, and we go into anaerobic metabolism. In this state, the muscles begin to accumulate lactate and other metabolites, and the muscle is infused with blood. Bodybuilders call this the 'pump'. This triggers protein synthesis and the subsequent building of new muscle tissue.

To achieve the desired level of metabolic stress, you need to include higher rep sets. Going up to 20 reps will achieve the pump effect needed. You can also achieve the peak contractions needed for maximum blood flow with isometrics.

Next up in the strength training pyramid is Progression.

PROGRESSION

To continue seeing benefits for your strength training investment, you need to be making the workout progressively harder. This can be done by:

- Increasing the resistance
- Increasing the repetitions

Let's say that you are doing the dumbbell curl with a weight that allows you to do 8 repetitions with good form. Each succeeding workout push yourself to perform an extra repetition without losing your good technique. When, after a period of weeks, you are able to do 12 reps with the weight that you started out doing 8 reps with, increase the weight slightly and drop back to 8 reps. You can continue progressing in this manner without limit.

Keep in mind that our strength can fluctuate for no apparent reason. Sometimes you may turn up for your workout and not be able to push past your previous limits. That's ok - so long as you are pushing yourself to the best of your ability on that day.

The penultimate level of the strength training pyramid considers rest intervals and tempo.

REST INTERVALS / TEMPO

The rest intervals between each set that you do should allow you to sufficiently recover from the previous set so that you are able to exert maximum force on the upcoming set. Of course, there will naturally be a cumulative muscle fatigue effect which cannot be avoided. You also want to build on the intensity of the last set to create a stair step stress effect on the muscle. All of this requires fine balancing of the ideal rest between sets time. Much research has gone into this subject. The consensus is that for maximum strength and muscle stimulation effect, you should rest for between 60-90 seconds per set.

Tempo relates to the speed with which you perform an exercise. You should perform your reps with a moderate tempo under control and without the use of any momentum.

A couple of factors that relate directly to your training tempo are time under tension and concentric / eccentric reps.

Time Under Tension

Time under tension, or TUT, refers to the total amount of time that a muscle is kept under tension in a set. When you incorporate TUT training in your workout, you prolong the time that your muscle is under tension in a rep by holding, or sometimes bouncing slightly, in the contracted position. TUT can also involve taking twice as long on the eccentric phase of the exercise than on the concentric phase. According to a 2016 study, doubling the length of the eccentric phase may result in greater muscle growth.

Concentric / Eccentric Reps

A repetition can be broken down into three parts; the lifting and the lowering portions, and the transition between them. The lifting part of the rep is known as the concentric, or positive, part, while the lowering portion is known as the eccentric or negative part.

Using the example of bicep curls, the lifting part where you curl the weight from your thighs to your shoulders is the concentric portion of the rep. The lowering part where you return to the start position is the eccentric portion. You are stronger during the eccentric part of the rep so that you can lower more weight than you can lift.

Research has shown that both the concentric and eccentric parts of the rep is beneficial to strength and muscle gains. You should take slightly longer on the eccentric part of the rep.

You should aim to follow a 2:1:3 tempo for best results. This means that you take 2 seconds to lift the weight (concentric), 1 second to hold in the peak contracted transition position and three seconds to lower the weight (eccentric).

A note on muscle damage - an effective muscle building workout will cause microtears in the muscle tissue. This will lead to soreness the next day and be the catalyst for protein synthesis. But we don't want to cause too much muscle damage, or all of the protein synthesis will go towards rebuilding old muscle rather than creating new muscle.

As you can handle a resistance that is as much as 20 percent heavier than you could on a concentric rep, when contracting your muscle concentrically, focusing on your eccentric reps is a great way to enhance muscle damage. You can also decrease the speed of the eccentric part of the rep, going from 2 to 4 seconds to complete the movement (i.e., increasing the TUT).

However, if you are focusing on eccentrics, the frequency of workouts must allow sufficient time for the muscles to recover from the stress imposed by your strength training session. Sufficient time is needed for the microtears in the muscle to repair themselves with the aid of the nutrients that you put into your body after the workout. That way they will grow back bigger and stronger than they were before your training session.

Finally, the apex of the strength training pyramid involves us thinking about the details of the program.

SPECIFICS/ DETAILS

The specifics and details relate to any customization of the program that are geared toward your specific goals and needs. For example, if you have a specific area of weakness, such as in the hamstrings, you might work them more than your quads in order to balance the strength between opposing muscle groups.

STRENGTH TRAINING IN PRACTICE

Society has fed us on the notion that older people have completely unique exercise requirements than younger people. That is completely false. Being older doesn't change much about your body's physiological needs for exercise. The muscles are still in the same place, they still have the same origin and insertion points, and they still respond in the same way to the stress of strength training.

The only difference between a 25-year-old and 55-year-old is that the 55-year old's body has had an extra 30 years to decondition itself. During this time, if he or she has not been doing strength training, his muscles will have atrophied. Yet, both the 25 and the 55-year-old require the same physiological mechanism to get stronger and build muscle. The 25-year-old and the 55-year-old both need to follow the same safety precautions, though the older person has a greater need to adhere to them.

All strength trainers need to perform biomechanically correct movements that allows them to move the muscle through a full range of motion. The exercise must also be done in such a way that it properly tracks joint and muscle function. The exercise must also be done in such a way that it properly controls the forces brought to bear on the muscles, joints and connective tissues.

One key issue to avoid at any age, but especially when you get past your 40th birthday, is excessive spinal loading. One of the main exercises in the gym that causes excessive spinal loading is the barbell squat. This exercise involves a tremendous amount of spinal compression due to the heavy weight that sits at the top of the spinal column. That load overloads the erector spinae and can cause irreparable disc damage. A far safer and wiser option, especially for older people, is to perform the cable or goblet version of the squat movement.

Perform the cable squat by setting a double pulley cable machine to its lowest pulley setting. Face the machine and grab the handles, stepping back about half a meter from the weight stacks so that your arms are fully extended. Try to stay upright as you squat down to a full squat position and then push through your heels to return to the start position. You will feel this movement directly working in the quadriceps, without compromising your spine.

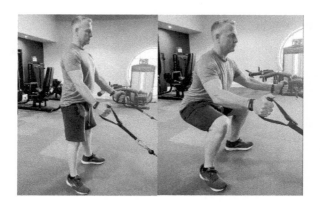

As an older exerciser, your focus needs to be on controlling the weight that you are using. That may require reducing the weight. Too many people, especially those who exercise in a commercial gym, work out to impress others or to achieve a certain weightlifting goal. That is not the way to get results. Never let the desire to go heavy get in the way of proper exercise form.

Keep in mind that your muscles have no idea what the number is on the side of the weight. All it knows is how much stress is being applied to it. Using a weight that is correct for your ability, you can control for the desired number of reps. This will place more stress on the muscle - and therefore generate more results - than a weight that is too heavy, requiring you to use momentum and the assistance of other muscle groups to get the weight up. By using lighter weight and slowly down the eccentric (negative) part of the movement you will be amazed at the results.

As an older trainer you should also focus on developing the mind muscle connection. Concentrate on how the muscle feels during the movement. See the muscle fibers expanding and contracting in your mind's eye and become attuned to the feel of that movement. This will allow you to get the maximum benefit out of every rep. It will also allow you to develop joint stability and muscle control.

When you were younger you may have emphasized working the 'show' muscles of the body, such as the biceps and chest, abs and glute muscles. As you get older, however, you need to train more wisely. That means not neglecting any of the major muscles of the body. Any body part that is neglected will become your weak link.

You need to be training each of the following body parts as equally as possible:

- Pectorals
- Latissimus Dorsi
- Deltoids
- Trapezius
- Rhomboids
- Rotator Cuff
- Biceps
- Triceps
- Forearms
- Abdominals and Obliques

- Erector Spinae
- Quadriceps
- Glutes
- Hamstrings
- Calves

SAMPLE WORKOUTS.

The following strength training workouts are designed for a person who has not done any regular strength training before or who is getting back into a resistance training routine. You will need access to a gym for these workouts. This is a two-day split, so that the person is training half the body one day and the other half of the body the next day. The emphasis for the first couple of workouts is to learn the proper exercise motion and establish the mind muscle connection that we have spoken about. You should also be experimenting to find the correct weight for the repetitions you are performing. From your third session onward, you should be working to increase the intensity of each workout by increasing the reps or the resistance.

On each successive set that you perform for an exercise, increase the weight slightly.

WARMING UP / COOLING DOWN

You must warm-up before every workout. Doing so will raise your body temperature, increase the mobility of your joints, increase blood flow and get you mentally primed.

Begin each workout with 3- 5 minutes of light cardio. If you don't have access to an exercise bike or treadmill, you can simply jog around your garden/ outdoor space. Or jog on the spot for 60 seconds, perform jumping jacks for 30 seconds, followed by high knees for another 30 seconds and repeat 2-3 times.

Next, do some dynamic stretching specifically to the body parts you will be working on. These could include arm circles, leg swings, trunk circles, bodyweight squats, or lunges. We will explore this further in the Mobility chapter.

After the workout, you should do static stretching, which we shall explore further in the flexibility chapter. I also recommend using a foam roller to perform a self-myofascial release massage either pre and/or post workout. This simply involves placing the roller between the muscle group you wish to work and the floor or a wall. You then roll back and forth to apply pressure to the muscle. The degree to which you push down on the roller dictates how deeply you penetrate the muscle tissue. We will also explore this further in the Mobility chapter.

Monday Workout – Upper Body

Pectorals, Latissimus Dorsi, Rhomboids, Trapezius, Deltoids, Rotator Cuff, Biceps, Triceps, Forearms

Exercise	Sets	Repetitions	Rest Between Sets
Decline Dumbbell Press	5	20/15/10/8/8	60- 90 seconds
One Arm Lat Pull In	5	20/15/10/8/8	60-90 seconds
Shrugs	4	20/15/10/8	60-90 seconds
Rear Delt Cable Extension	4	20/15/10/8	60-90 seconds
Cable Deltoid Press	4	20/15/10/8	60-90 seconds
Decline Dumbbell Triceps Extension	4	20/15/10/8	60-90 seconds
Alternate Dumbbell Curl	4	20/16/10/8	60-90 seconds
Barbell Wrist Curl	3	20/15/10	60-90 seconds

Tuesday Workout – Lower Body and Core

Quadriceps, Glutes, Hamstrings, Calves, Abdominals, Obliques, Erector Spinae

Exercise	Sets	Repetitions	Rest Between Sets
Cable or Goblet Squat	5	20/15/10/8/8	60-90 seconds
Barbell Hip Thrusts or Glute kickback machine	5	20/15/10/8/8	60-90 seconds
Alternative Dumbbell Reverse Lunges	4	20,16,10,8	60-90 seconds
Seated Leg Curl	4	20/15/10/8	60-90 seconds
Seated or Standing Calf Raise	4	25/20/15/10	60-90 seconds
Cable Crunch	3	25/20/15	60-90 seconds
Cable Torso Rotation	3	15/15/15	60-90 seconds
Seated Torso Extension	3	25/20/15	60-90 seconds

SUMMARY

Strength training will form the main foundation of your total fitness program. Make it your goal to perfect your exercise form, really feeling the working muscles and concentrating on moving through a full range of motion. Challenge yourself to progressively increase the resistance you are working with so as to make consistent improvement in your strength and muscle mass. Do these things week in and week out, and you will be amazed at how much stronger, more muscular, energetic and vibrant you will look and feel.

Now it's time to discover how the next foundation will play its vital role in your health and fitness journey...

4

FLEXIBILITY - STRETCH TO IMPRESS

I f you've ever marveled at the ability of children to put their feet behind their head or do the splits and then struggled to bend down to tie your shoes, you have become painfully aware of the effect that age has on flexibility. When we move into our 40s, we start to begin to notice that the things we used to take for granted are just that little bit more difficult to perform. These changes are subtle but there will come a point when you'll realize just how much flexibility you've lost.

The good news is that, while you may have lost some flexibility, it is not that difficult to find it again. Understanding what flexibility is, the different forms it takes, and when you should do each one is the key to reclaiming the flexibility of your youth.

WHAT IS FLEXIBILITY?

Flexibility is the ability of your joints to move freely through their complete range of motion. Flexibility training helps to improve the range of motion of your muscles.

If you don't have good flexibility, such everyday activities as getting out of bed, bending down to pick up a child or squatting down to lift a heavy or light object can become more demanding. A lack of adequate flexibility can also impair your athletic ability, as you will be unable to reach the full potential, strength and power of your muscles.

FLEXIBILITY BENEFITS

Increased Range of Motion: Range of motion is the distance and direction your joints can move. Consistent flexibility training will increase the range of motion of your joints and muscles. It does this by lengthening the muscles and opening the joints. As a result, you'll be able to stretch further in all directions while remaining pain free.

Decreased Risk of Injury: People with flexible muscles are less likely to become injured during physical activity.

Reduced Muscle Soreness: Flexibility training helps to reduce muscle soreness after you exercise. When you stretch after your workout, you keep your muscles loose and relaxed.

Improved Athletic Performance: When your joint and muscles are flexible, you use less energy in motion. This makes you more efficient, improving your performance.

WHY WE BECOME LESS FLEXIBLE WITH AGE

When most people enter their 40s, they notice a marked drop off in their flexibility. At the same time, their joints become achy. That's because, as we age, our ligaments are not as flexible as they used to be. The amount of synovial fluid inside the joints diminishes and the cartilage becomes thinner. This appears to be most prevalent around the hips and knees.

As we age, the tissue that surrounds our joints also thickens. This contributes to a lack of flexibility. The loss of muscle mass and the associated strength decline is another contributor to reduced flexibility as we age. In tandem with age related muscle loss, many people accumulate more stored body fat as they age, further exacerbating the lack of flexibility problem.

A simple thing we can all do to improve our flexibility is to drink more water. This will increase the lubrication of the joints, helping to offset the natural loss of synovial fluid that occurred with aging. Enhancing joint movement through exercise will also help to reverse cartilage shrinkage and increase mobility.

MOST COMMON FLEXIBILITY ISSUES FOR THE ELDERLY

Limited flexibility most commonly evidences itself in the elderly with reduced movement in the hips and spine. This is the cause of chronic and ongoing pain for millions of people. Though back pain can have a number of root causes, impaired flexibility in the hamstrings, glutes and hip flexors is often a major contributing factor.

When a person has tight hamstrings, these muscles will unnaturally pull the pelvis downward. This will result in lower back tension and soreness.

The hip flexor muscles are connected to the leg bones (femur or tibia) and the hip joint. They allow the knee to lift the thigh up and to the sides. The three main hip flexor muscles are the:

- Iliopsoas
- Sartorius
- Rectus Femoris

When we are in a sedentary, seated position for hours on end, our hips maintain a flexed position. The lack of movement of the hip flexors causes them cumulatively to shorten and shrink. Tightness in muscles such as the iliopsoas will cause you to compress your spine and tilt your pelvis forward - again leading to tension in the lower back.

The piriformis muscle is situated in the buttocks above the hip joint. It assists the hip flexors to lift and moves the thighs away from the body. Lack of flexibility can lead to piriformis syndrome, which is characterized by numbness and pain in the buttocks. As a result of the piriformis muscle pressing down on the sciatic nerve, many people also experience pain running down each leg, which is known as sciatica.

GENDER DIFFERENCES

Women naturally have greater hip flexibility than men do. This results from a greater preponderance of estrogenic hormones which are designed to prepare the female body for the rigors of childbirth. As a result, women have enhanced hip bone mobility through the pelvis, as well as better mobility through the tailbone. They also have a wider and more circular pelvis than men.

The bone and muscle changes that occur in females during puberty make their lower body joints less stable than male joints. One result of this is that, when resistance is applied to the quads and knees (such as when doing the squat), the knees tend to buckle inward.

Women also naturally have better shoulder joint mobility, especially through the anterior (front) deltoid's range of motion.

TYPES OF STRETCHING

Dynamic Stretching

It has become increasingly popular over recent years, as studies have shown the negative effects of static stretching on training performance before exercise. Dynamic stretching involves speed of movement, momentum and active muscular effort to perform a stretch. Often the stretch mimics or is closely linked to the upcoming athletic performance.

It is good to include some dynamic stretching in your warmup routine, regardless of the type of exercise you are doing, as it is a good way to reduce tightness in the muscles while upping the core temperature of the body and enhancing the range of motion around your joints. It also prepares your body for the specific demands of the activity that you will be performing during your training session. Examples of dynamic stretches include walking knee hugs, side lunges, ankle and wrist rotations, leg swings and torso twists. We shall explore this further in the next chapter.

Static Stretching

Static stretching, also known as isometric stretching, involves extending a muscle until you feel a gentle stretch. This is the best form of stretching to improve flexibility and is ideally done immediately after your strength training workout. You can also perform a separate static stretching session later in the day, taking more time to stretch for longer. If you are completing a separate stretching session, you should, as always, warm up your body for a few minutes before.

PNF Stretching

Proprioceptive Neuromuscular Facilitation (PNF) is an adaptation of static stretching. It involves both stretching and contracting the target muscle group. It is extremely effective at improving flexibility and increasing range of motion.

PNF stretching relies on the stretch reflex of the myotendinous unit by activating mechanoreceptors within the muscle called muscle spindle units and Golgi tendon organs. Muscle spindles help to regulate overall muscle length and tone by activating gamma motor neurons by way of the stretch reflex.

The initial isometric contraction (hold) phase of the PNF stretch lasts for 10 seconds at 40 percent maximal contraction. The muscle then relaxes into a passive stretch for 30 seconds. You repeat this 4 times then, on the 5th contraction, you hold the position for 15 seconds. With each repetition you slightly increase the stretch position.

Ballistic Stretching

Ballistic stretching involves stretching a muscle to where you feel a gentle stretch and then bouncing to extend the stretch even further. This form of stretching is NOT recommended as it carries a risk of injury to the muscle.

FLEXIBILITY TESTING

Before you begin a stretching program, you should determine your current level of flexibility. Retest every 8 weeks to gauge your progress.

Precede your tests with 5 minutes of light cardio exercise such as skipping or light running to ensure your muscles are warm.

Here are 4 examples:

Modified Sit & Reach Test

Lower Back and Hamstring Flexibility

For this test you will need a 30cm high box and a one meter rule.

Sit with your back against a wall and your legs outstretched and together. Have a friend position the box against your feet. Keeping your shoulder blades against the wall and your knees straight, stretch your arms forward. Have your friend put the meter rule on the box and move it forward until the end touches your fingertips. This is your zero point.

Now stretch forward as far as possible without bending your knees. Have your friend record the distance of your stretch on the meter rule. Do not bounce or jerk during the stretch.

Repeat the test three times and take the average.

Trunk Rotation Test

Trunk & Shoulder Flexibility

For this test you will need a wall and a piece of chalk.

Stand in front of a wall and mark a vertical line on it. Stand facing away from the wall in front of the line, arm's length away from it. Extend your arms in front of your torso. Now twist your torso to the left and touch the wall behind you with your fingertips. Mark this point with the chalk. Measure the distance from the line. A point before the line is a negative score and a point after the line is a positive score.

Repeat on the right side and then take the average of the two scores.

Groin Flexibility Test

Groin Flexibility

You will need a ruler for this test.

Sit on the floor with knees bent, and your legs together with feet flat on the floor. Keeping your feet together, drop your knees down to the sides. Now grab your feet with both hands and pull your ankles toward your body. Have a friend measure the distance between your heels and your groin.

Thomas test

Hip Flexibility

You will need a ruler for this test.

Lie supine (on your back) on a table with both lower legs hanging off the end (knees flexed). Bring your right knee towards your chest and hold just below the knee with both hands. Keep your lower back flat on the table if you can. If there is no tightness in the left hip, the leg will remain flat on the table. If there is tightness, then the left leg will rise off the table. Ask a friend to use the ruler to measure how high your left leg is off the table. Repeat on the other leg. Here are 4 things to look out for:

- Increased lumbar lordosis (arch of the lower back) could mean tight hip flexors.
- If you are unable to bring the hip into full extension so it rests in the air could mean tight hip flexors.
- If you are unable to bring the knee to 90 degree flexion and hold it in place could mean tight quadriceps.
- If your knee drifts to the side into hip abduction, this could also mean a tight TFL muscle.

STRETCHING RECOMMENDATIONS

- The American College of Sports Medicine (ACSM)

recommends flexibility exercises for all of the major muscle-tendon groups - neck, shoulders, trunk, lower back, hips, legs, ankles - 2-3 times per week.

- Spend up to 60 seconds on each stretch; if you can only hold the stretch for 20 seconds, repeat the stretch three times.
- Never bounce into a stretch.
- Perform dynamic stretches before your workout.
- Perform static stretching after your workout.
- If you are doing a separate stretching session, do a 5 minute warm up of cardio and dynamic stretches.

16 GREAT STATIC STRETCHES

N.B. Always stretch both sides for the same amount of time!

Neck Stretch

Bend your head forward so that your chin touches your upper chest. Bend your head backwards so that you are looking at the ceiling. Bend your head to the left side, trying to get your ear to touch your shoulder. Repeat this on the right side. Hold for 60 seconds each.

Latissimus Dorsi Stretch

Place both hands face down on a fence, ledge or mantel. Bending at the waist, let your body drop down while keeping your knees slightly bent and arms straight out in front of you. Hold this gentle stretch for 60 seconds.

Spinal Stretch

Start by kneeling on your hands and knees. Push your hips back, so your pelvis sinks between your knees and your head rests on the floor. Extend your hands out as far as you can in front of you. Hold for 60 seconds.

Oblique Stretch

Standing - Lean to the right, keeping your left arm straight over your head, and right arm on your hip. Hold for 60 seconds.

Arms, Shoulders & Chest Stretch

Grab a towel at both ends while keeping your arms straight. Without bending your arms, raise the towel over your head and behind your back. Hold the towel behind your back for 60 seconds.

Pectoral Stretch

Standing – Place your right forearm onto a door frame so that your fingertips are pointing toward the ceiling. Your upper arm should be at shoulder height with your elbow bent at 90 degrees. Place your right foot forward and rotate your torso away from the frame. Hold for 60 seconds and repeat with the left arm.

Forearm & Wrist Stretch

Get down on your hands and knees. Turn your hands outwards until your thumbs are on the outside and your fingers are pointed towards your knees. Keeping your arms straight, start to lean backwards until you feel an easy stretch in your forearms. Hold for 60 seconds.

Hip Flexor Stretch

Start by kneeling on a mat, then place your right foot forward so that you have a 90-degree angle at the hip and knee. The left knee should remain on the floor, aligned underneath the left hip. Place your hands on the right knee for support (if needed). Keeping the torso upright, slightly tuck your pelvis under. Slowly lean forward until you feel a comfortable stretch in front of your left hip. Hold for 60 seconds.

Quad Stretch

Standing - Hold your foot at the lace part of your shoe (not your ankle), bring it behind your body and tuck your pelvis under so your tailbone is pointing at the wall in front of you (a posterior tilt). Try and get your heel to touch your glute without letting your knee swing out to the side. Hold for 60 seconds.

Hamstring Stretch

Standing - With your feet hip width apart, place your right leg forward so your right heel is just in front of your left toe. Keeping your right leg straight, place your hands on your left knee and bend the knee. With a straight back, gently lean forward resting your weight on your bent leg. Hold for 60 seconds.

Glute Stretch

Sit on a chair and cross your right ankle just above your left knee. Place your hands on the inner side of your right knee, lean forward slightly and apply gentle pressure. Hold for 60 seconds.

Groin Stretch

Sit on the floor with the soles of your feet together while grabbing them with your hands. Your heels should be a comfortable distance (for you) from your crotch. Gently pull yourself forward, keeping your back straight, until you feel an easy stretch in your groin. Hold for 60 seconds.

Abductor Stretch

Standing - lean forward and grab onto a chair for balance. Cross one foot behind the other and slide that foot away from your body, keeping your legs straight. Slowly bend your front leg to lower your body. Hold for 60 seconds.

Calf Stretch I

Position the ball of your foot on the edge of a stair. Your other foot should be completely on the stair and you may wish to grab a railing or wall for balance. Lower the heel of your foot below the stair level. Hold for 60 seconds.

Calf Stretch II

Stand facing a wall and place your palms on it in line with your chest. Step your right leg back so that it is fully extended with your left knee slightly bent. Now lean forward to the wall, keeping your back foot completely on the floor. You should feel the stretch through your calf muscle. Hold for 60 seconds.

The World's Greatest Stretch

This stretch does indeed live up to its moniker, as it stretches almost every major muscle group in some way. It has been modified over the years and you can find numerous variations online. Here is a relatively easy version to follow:

1. Standing hip width apart, lunge forward with your right leg and put your left hand on the ground opposite the right leg. You will now be in a balanced half kneeling or exaggerated sprint position. Your front (right) knee should be directly above your ankle and back (left) ankle behind your toe.
2. Keeping your left leg as straight as you can, lower your right forearm to the ground and hold for 10 seconds.

3. Keeping your hips still and in line with your back (left) leg, extend your right arm up to 90 degrees towards the ceiling, rotating your torso. Look up and hold for 10 seconds. Try to keep your back foot still as you rotate.

4. Bring your right arm down and rotate underneath your torso to the left. Hold for 10 seconds.

Repeat this action 10 times and switch sides.

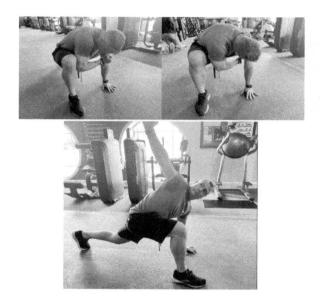

YOGA FOR FLEXIBILITY

Yoga is an all-encompassing term which describes a system of wellbeing that originated in ancient India. Yoga embraces breathing exercises, relaxation and meditation techniques and physical movement. In terms of flexibility improvement, it is *hatha,* or physical yoga that is our focus.

Yoga is a smart choice for people wanting to improve their flexibility. It provides a gentle journey through your comfort zone, without forcing your body. Being a low impact form of exercise, yoga is accessible to all people, be they seasoned athletes or couch potatoes.

Yoga provides a holistic approach to stretching. Conventional stretching stretches one muscle group at a time. However, hatha yoga unites the person, synchronizing the body, the breath and the mind.

Yoga will make you more flexible, which will, in turn, make you more agile. And, a more agile body is a more balanced, stronger body. Agility refers to the body's ability to change direction and position of the body fluidly without physical or mental strain. The bending, rotating and pivoting involved in yoga will keep you agile all day long.

Your body balance and proprioception, which relates to your awareness of your body's position in space, are also heightened by yoga training.

Yoga Positioning

Body positioning is integral to successful yoga practice. There are three parts to every yoga pose:

1. Movement into the pose
2. Stillness while holding the pose
3. Movement out of the pose

Each of these areas are equally important. Unless your positioning is on point, you are likely to cause injury to your muscles and joints.

As a beginner, you need to perfect your yoga positioning. How can you do it?

I suggest joining a yoga studio for a month in order to learn the proper technique.

SUMMARY

We have now discovered the issues that are inherent with a lack of flexibility as we age, but more importantly, the benefits of exercise and strategies as simple as hydration for improving our flexibility. You can perform dynamic stretches at the beginning of a workout to help your muscles warm up; static stretches at the end of a gym session, which will help your muscles recover from exercise; and also longer stretching sessions on their own at home when you are watching TV, or listening to music or audiobooks. The key is to make sure that however you do it, you are stretching regularly and gently. Flexibility does take time to achieve and requires a lot of patience, but you will get there with time! The key, as with all my 7 foundations, is consistency. In our next chapter we will explore another key foundation of total fitness that flexibility is essential to help maintain. Luckily for us, this next foundation is more dynamic, and in my opinion can be a lot of fun to train.

Let's get moving...

5

MOBILITY - MOVE IT OR LOSE IT!

L oss of mobility is one of the classic signs of aging. In fact, it's a stereotype of people over the age of 60. They are expected to be mobility challenged, to stumble and fall at the slightest obstacle. Yet, as we discovered earlier, loss of mobility is not an inevitable sign of aging. Mobility, the ability to move your body freely through a range of motion without pain, can be maintained and even enhanced by maintaining daily exercise habits, controlling your weight and following a balanced diet.

THE IMPORTANCE OF MOBILITY

A mobile person is able to maintain control over the contraction of their muscles throughout the whole of a joint movement. For instance, when you straighten out your elbow and then bend it so that your fist comes up to your shoulder, you are flexing and extending the elbow joint by contracting the biceps muscles. If you are mobile, your muscles will be strong and flexible enough to move the joint through its whole range of motion in a controlled manner, as well as to stop and hold the movement at any given point. Essentially, being mobile means that you have total control over your joints and muscles.

When you establish a base of mobility, you are able to build strength and explosiveness and realize your potential in any exercise or sporting pursuit that you put your mind to. In fact, mobility underpins all of the benefits of strength training that were detailed in the previous chapter. If you are lacking in mobility, you will struggle to perform the strength training exercises that were laid out in that chapter. It makes sense, then, to follow a mobility enhancement routine in tandem with your strength training.

Lack of mobility is a major contributor to falls in the elderly. Combine this with loss of muscular strength, stability and flexibility and it's not hard to understand why falls have become the leading cause of traumatic death over the age of 65 in the United States. Yet, the combination of mobility and strength training will dramatically offset the lack of mobility and subsequent balance problems that many people think are part and parcel of getting older.

People who are able to maintain a high level of mobility as they move into their 60s and 70s experience a much greater sense of freedom, independence and overall quality of life. In contrast, those who suffer from limited mobility experience pain every time they move a muscle and have to put up with creaky joints. They can't help but feel that their zest for life and energy is slowly but consistently being drained away.

Importantly, elderly people who have a good level of mobility are able to live independently for longer. They are able to carry out their everyday tasks without assistance, cook for themselves, play with their grandkids, and enjoy leisure activities outside of the home. This has a huge psychological benefit, allowing them to stay connected, feel part of things and really enjoy their golden years and everything that they have to offer.

Why We Become Less Mobile As We Age

Loss of mobility as we age is a combination of the following factors:

- Age related muscle loss ('sarcopenia')
- Loss of bone mass
- Reduction in range of joint motion
- Accumulation of body fat
- Lack of physical movement
- Poor dietary habits

As we think about each of these factors, we realize that they can all be offset through our lifestyle habits. Sure, the first three factors are a natural part of aging. We will all lose between 3-8 percent of our muscle mass every decade after the age of 30; by the age of 40, each of us will begin to lose joint movement - our hip joint flexion will decrease by 6-7 degrees per decade, and concurrently our shoulder range of motion will go down by 5-6 degrees. Yet, the right type of strength and mobility exercises can help to offset those natural losses. There are many thousands of examples of men and women in their 40s, 50s and 60s who are stronger, have more muscle AND greater mobility than they did in their 20s and 30s.

Obesity is a major risk factor for the loss of mobility. An obese person puts far greater demands on his skeletal muscles than a healthy weight person does. High levels of adipose tissue (fat) have also been associated with reduced functional muscle ability and strength. Lack of flexibility and control over muscles is also more readily seen among overweight individuals.

TYPICAL MOBILITY ISSUES

Mobility problems usually manifest themselves as difficulty with walking or maintaining a healthy posture. Balance issues are also common with people as they age. In fact, this is the number one reason that elderly people make appointments to see their doctor. Not all balance issues, however, are mobility related. Vertigo, inner ear problems and nerve conditions may also be at the root of the problem.

Postural problems that are linked to lack of mobility typically exacerbate with age. When you are standing with a normal posture your spine will have a normal forward curvature. This is called 'kyphosis'. This is matched by reverse curvature ('lordosis') in the cervical and lumbar spine. These natural curvatures allow us to sit up and stand with ideal positioning.

Postural problems occur when we develop an exaggerated forward curvature of the upper spine. This has become a huge problem in recent decades as a result of our computer dominant lifestyles. Most people spend more than an hour each day hunched over some form of technology nowadays. The excessive forward curvature that develops as a result is known as 'hyperkyphosis'.

Something as simple as doing daily scapular retractions can be a huge help! You can do these by sitting or standing upright and squeezing your shoulder blades down and back so they move closer together. This will also make your chest look bigger which is an extra bonus! Just be careful not to lean back as it will hyperextend your lumbar spine (lower back). You can modify this by extending your elbows and fingers to create a mountain pose. This is the complete opposite of what we do in our day to day lives as you are focusing on thoracic extension rather than flexion.

IMPROVING YOUR MOBILITY

Improving your mobility should be something that fits seamlessly into your exercise program. In other words, it doesn't have to be a separate workout in its own right (though it can be) but, rather, can be included as an extension of your strength training workout. Mobility training should include the following elements:

- Myofascial tissue massage to release and loosen muscles
- Dynamic stretching
- Mobility drills

Perform your mobility work as part of your warm-up to your strength training session. The total duration of your mobility warm-up should ideally be around 10 minutes.

SELF MYOFASCIAL RELEASE

Self-Myofascial Release (SMR) is a form of self-massage which has become hugely popular among runners and exercise enthusiasts due to its ease of application and immediacy of result. SMR involves alleviating soft-tissue stiffness and pain hot spots with a form of self-massage. It has also proven to be a great post-workout recovery aid.

SMR makes use of a simple massage aid, such as a foam roller or massage ball, to manipulate and put pressure on muscle sore spots. In addition to its rehabilitative ability SMR has been shown to improve flexibility and exercise performance.

To understand how SMR manages to achieve its quite remarkable outcomes with such a seemingly simple procedure, we need to delve into the mysteries of the body's kinetic chain. The kinetic chain refers to the interconnected soft tissue, neural and articular systems. If any one of these systems is not working optimally, the other systems compensate by working harder. If left unchecked, this will lead to tissue overload, fatigue, pain and restricted mobility.

SMR works on the two neural receptors that are found in your muscles, the muscle spindle and the golgi tendon organ. Muscle spindles, located parallel to muscle fibers, send messages to the central nervous system about fiber length changes as a result of injury, which triggers the myotatic stretch reflex. The result? Pain.

Golgi tendon organ overstimulation can likewise lead to inhibited movement and soreness. Soft tissue massage focused on these receptors provides immediate relief from pain, restores normal fiber length and improves function.

Using a Foam Roller

A foam roller is a cylindrical piece of high density foam. The most basic form is a flat edged EPE soft roller. Trigger Point Grid Foam rollers are firmer and feature grooves, indentations and protrusions that allow you to penetrate your trigger points.

Find an open space that allows freedom of movement. Place the roller on the floor and position your body so that the area of focus is on top of the roller. The pressure that massages the affected area will be provided by your body.

Gently roll your body back and forth over the roller. Your focus should be on areas of tightness and those that have a reduced range of motion - if you feel a tight spot, hold the stretch there for a few seconds. Control this pressure by adjusting the amount of bodyweight that you place on the roller. You can use your hands and feet to offset the weight as needed.

Here are most effective foam rolling moves for your major muscle groups:

Quadriceps

Rest one leg on the ground and place the other thigh over the edge of the foam roller, just above the knee. Support your body on your palms and elbows. Now roll the thigh up and down by pushing your hips back. As you roll, place pressure on all four of the quadriceps muscles to emphasize that area.

Hamstrings

Sit on the floor with the foam roller resting under one hamstring just above the knee. Support your body by resting your palms on the floor behind you. Now move up and down the roller from your knees to your hips by pushing your hips back and forth.

Calves

Sit on the floor with the foam roller resting under one calf just below the knee. Support your body by resting your palms on the floor behind you. Now move up and down the roller from your knee to your ankle by pushing your hips back and forth.

IT Band/TFL

Lie on the floor sideways with one hip resting on the foam roller. Bend your other knee with the sole of your foot on the floor. Start rolling from the bottom of the thigh, just above your knee, and come up to the outer part of the hip.

Back

Lie on the floor with the foam roller under your shoulder blades. Roll up and down your back with slow, smooth movements. Try to avoid going any lower than your ribs as the lower back is a more vulnerable area. If you have a specific trigger point area in your back, you may want to use a tennis ball to apply direct pressure to that area. You can also do this standing against a wall. This is particularly useful for the lower back as you are able to better control the pressure.

Chest

Lie face down on the foam roller, with it directly underneath your sternum (breastplate) and orientated so it points towards your head. With your arm out to the side, you can then roller down the length of the pectoral muscles from the sternum to your armpit. This stretch is most useful for men - if you are a woman and you find this impractical, you can use a tennis ball against a wall and apply pressure point massage as needed.

DYNAMIC STRETCHING

Dynamic stretching involves moving your muscles through their full range of motion. Dynamic stretches often simulate the resistance moves that are part of the workout to come, such as doing bodyweight squats or lunges.

Here is a 5 move dynamic stretching routine that will enhance your mobility ahead of your workout:

Bodyweight Squats w/high knees x 10

Stand with your feet shoulder width apart and your arms extended out in front of you. Maintain a neutral spine, then hinge from the hips to lower down into a parallel squat position. Push through the heels to return to the start position. You can also add in alternate high knees or mini kicks as a good modification.

Overhead Twisting Reverse Lunge x 5 (each side)

From the same starting position, take a large step backwards with your left leg and lower down into a lunge position. Now, keeping your arms straight overhead, twist your torso to the right then back to the center. Push back through the right thigh to return to the start position. After 5 reps, repeat on the right leg.

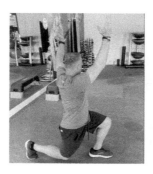

Superman x 10

Lie face down on an exercise mat with your body in an arched position so that your arms and feet are extended off the ground in a dish shape. Now arch up to full extension to bring your arms and feet up as high as possible. Lower and repeat.

Arm Circles x 20

Stand with your arms hanging at your sides. Now rotate from the shoulder joint to move your arms in wide circles at the sides of your body. Keep the elbows locked and concentrate on achieving a 360 degree range of motion.

World's Greatest Stretch – Dynamic x 10

As mentioned earlier in the flexibility chapter, The World's Greatest Stretch is one of the best all round stretches you can do. However this can also be done as a dynamic stretch by simply performing the steps outlined in chapter 4 but without holding the positions and alternating legs after each movement pattern. Two extra points to consider are

1. Try not to raise your hips when you switch legs.
2. Keep the flow of the movements smooth and focus on regulating your breathing.

MOBILITY DRILLS

Perform your mobility drills immediately after your dynamic stretching exercises. Perform 10 reps on each movement and then go straight into the next exercise. Once you've finished these, you'll be ready to get cracking with your training session!

Cat cows

Start on your hands and knees. Your knees directly under your hips and hands under your shoulders and with your spine neutral. As you inhale, move into cow pose by sticking your bum out and pressing your chest forward and allowing your upper back to sink. Lift your head looking forward and relax your shoulders away from your ears. Now exhale into cat pose by rounding your spine towards the ceiling and tucking in your tailbone. Relax your head and lower toward your chin. Repeat 10 times.

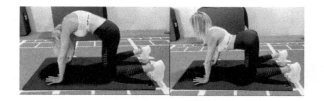

Walkouts

Stand with your feet hip to shoulder width apart and with good posture. Start to reach down to the ground with your hands and only bend your knees when you need to. This will give you a nice stretch in your hamstrings. Walk your hands out in front of you and keep your knees in line with your toes. Do this until you are in a perfect press up plank position. Hold for 2 seconds. Walk your hands back up towards your body to reverse the movement.

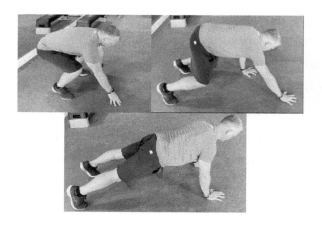

Standing hip circles

Standing tall, place your hands on your hips and feet slightly apart. Start to make a clockwise circular motion with your hips from left to right. Repeat 10 times then change direction.

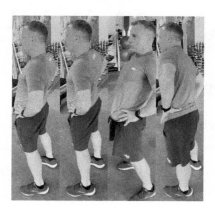

Leg swings

Stand sideways next to a wall, chair, door handle so you have plenty of room. Hold on with your hand next to the support and your outside hand on your hip. Keep your back upright and core engaged. Start to swing your furthest leg forward and back like a pendulum. Start slowly at first with a small range of motion and start to increase the range as the reps go up. You ideally want to get to a full range of motion at the hip but not so high that your back bends and your hip starts to rotate. 15 - 20 swings on each leg.

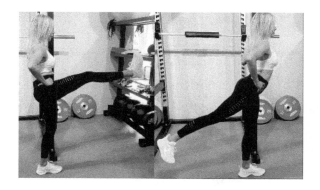

Lying Can openers

Lie on your right side and bend both knees. You can use a foam block in between the knees to help hip alignment and for your head to keep your neck neutral. Have both arms in front of your body with both hands touching. Keep your shoulder blades relaxed. Take your top (right) arm and rotate it round to the left till your back is as flat as possible. This action will rotate your torso. Try not to let your knees come off the ground or away from each other. Repeat 10 times then switch sides.

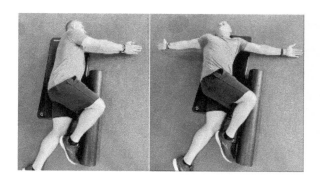

Dynamic crucifix

Lie down on a mat with straight legs and extend your arms out to the side so they are in line with your shoulders. Lift your right leg off the ground and bend your knee. Rotate it across your body to the left. Ideally your right hip should be facing the ceiling. Touch the floor with your right foot keeping your back as flat as you can. Switch directions and alternate 10 times.

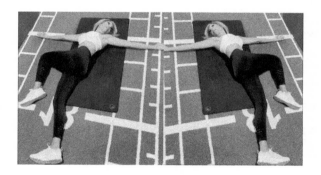

Fire hydrants

Start on your hands and knees. Your knees directly under your hips and hands under your shoulders and with your spine neutral and engaged. Keeping your torso and left leg completely still. Lift your right knee and raise it sideways away from your body. Bring it back to the starting position. Repeat 12 – 15 times.

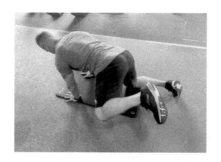

SUMMARY

Improving your mobility will do wonders for your enjoyment of life and your everyday functionality. Whether it's gardening, DIY or playing with your kids in the back yard. Getting there is not that difficult. In fact, the three-part routine (foam rolling, dynamic stretching and mobility drills) that we've covered in this chapter takes just a few minutes to complete. Add it in as part of your warm up before your strength training and you will be amazed at how much more fluid, mobile and free you will feel - try it and see for yourself! You can also perform these three aspects as a separate routine to wake you up in the morning. Your heart rate will increase while you do this, so it's a great jump start to the day.

In the next chapter, you will discover the benefits of yet another foundation and why its relationship with mobility is so important...

6

STABILITY - FINDING THE BALANCE

F alls are the number one cause of injury in people aged 60 and over. They can result in everything from pelvic fractures to head injuries, or even death. Scarily, 25% of people in this age bracket experience at least one fall per year.

But why do we fall?

Some falls are due to environmental factors (e.g. poor lighting, inappropriate footwear, or uneven surfaces), but the major issue for most people is one simple factor: a lack of stability. Stability describes our ability to control our body during movement. You can consider stability as the framework of a car. When you improve your body's stability system, you are developing a strong foundation to support your body's engine.

THE STABILITY-MOBILITY CONTINUUM

The joints of our body can move in three different planes of motion - the sagittal plane (flexion and extension, i.e. bending and straightening), the frontal plane (abduction and adduction, i.e. moving towards and away from the centerline of the body) and the transverse plane (rotation). Some joints are more mobile than others, moving in all three planes of motion (for example, our shoulders and hips). In comparison, joints like the knees and elbows are very stable, moving only in the sagittal plane. Your body needs a combination of mobile and stable joints in order to function effectively. In fact, the body alternates stable and mobile regions, which we can see if we look at the body as a chain from the ground up:

Ankle (mobile) > knee (stable) > hip (mobile) > lumbar region (stable) > thoracic region (mobile) > scapulothoracic joint (stable) > shoulder (mobile) > elbow (stable) > wrist (mobile)

In a normal situation, these stable and mobile regions work in tandem; however, if there is a change in any one of these regions, this has a knock-on effect on the rest of the chain and can result in an injury that is seemingly unrelated to the affected area! If a normally mobile joint has sub-optimal mobility, one of the more stable joints nearby will need to work to compensate to provide the missing movement.

For example, if your ankle lacks mobility, often the knee will compensate, resulting in knee pain. Similarly, if you lose mobility in your hips or thoracic region, this can lead to low back pain because the normally stable lumbar spine needs to provide additional movement so you can perform your everyday functions.

But it's not quite as black and white as pure 'mobile' and 'stable' regions. Every joint, no matter how mobile, needs some stability. And the opposite is also true - even very stable joints like the lumbar spine need to have some mobility! We should therefore consider every joint as located somewhere on a stability-mobility continuum.

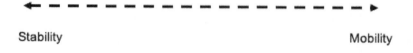

Each joint needs a specific balance of stability and mobility - even joints such as the shoulder and ankle that require large amounts of mobility need some stability to prevent pain and injury. In reality, our joints are placed on the stability-mobility continuum as shown below:

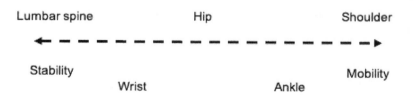

Ligament damage (such as a strain) can decrease the passive stability of a joint by making the ligaments more lax - this will improve mobility, but at the expense of necessary structural stability of the joint. This will put the joint at risk of further injury, and is one of the reasons that previous injury is one of the biggest predictors of future injury risk. It's also why it is so important for us to incorporate stability work into our exercise programming for total fitness.

KEEPING OUR BODY STABLE

There are three systems that help us keep our body stable: the proprioceptive, the visual, and the vestibular.

1. The Proprioceptive System. This system provides you with an awareness of where your body is in space and how much strength you need to perform a movement (for example, you need less force to open a crisp packet than to lift your grandchild into their car seat). This sense of perception and awareness of your body's position is crucial for you to engage effectively with your environment, as the information transmitted from sensory receptors to the brain dictates our muscle movement and actions.

2. The Visual System. We use our vision to detect information about our surroundings - for example, our

location, direction, speed of movement, obstacles, and the surface we are moving on.

3. The Vestibular System. This system is located within our inner ear, and consists of three fluid-filled channels. Movement of the neck causes movement of the fluid in these channels, which helps our brain detect our body position. It also allows us to determine the position and location of objects surrounding us.

As we age, the function of all of these systems becomes less efficient, leading to a gradual loss of stability with time. Reductions in the capacity of the visual and vestibular system come with the loss of vision and hearing often experienced with age, and they can also be a side-effect of disease or neurological conditions. The proprioceptive system also experiences declines, which impacts our movement as a whole - you are likely to walk slower, for example, if your body isn't sure where your foot is in relation to the ground. Together with the loss of muscle size and strength with age (known as sarcopenia), this drastically increases our risk of falling as we grow older.

Luckily for us, we now know that we can slow down this loss of muscle size and strength using resistance training. However, while strength training is key, it's not enough on its own. Unfortunately, there may not be much we can do to change the visual or vestibular systems, but we can supplement our training with exercises designed specifically to target the proprioceptive system. This will improve our stability through movement, reducing our risk of joint injuries, and as we get older, falls.

IMPROVING YOUR STABILITY

Now we know why stability is so important for reducing the risk of joint injuries and falls, we should consider how we can program exercise to improve our stability. There are two aspects of stability that need to be trained:

- Active Stability
- Passive Stability

Active stability relates to the body's mechanism for movement based on the signals that are sent from the brain. When you improve your active stability, you enhance your strength, mobility and stamina. We can improve our active stability by performing balance exercises.

Passive stability relates to the actual movement of your cartilage, bones and ligaments. We can consider these components to be the hardware of movement. Improving your passive stability through strength training will allow you to perform movement more fluidly.

Thinking about the regions that we described above as needing stability (i.e. knee, lower back, scapulothoracic region and elbow), we can see that the most important muscles you need to train to improve your body's stability are...

Lower Body

- The Core (abdominals and lumbar spine)
- The Quadriceps
- The Glutes

Upper Body

- Rotator cuff

Below are some simple exercises designed to target these muscle groups and train your joint stability. All you will need is an exercise band.

LOWER BODY

3 Types of Bridges - Targeting Hip Stability

1. Two Leg Bridge

Lie on your back with both knees bent and your feet flat on the floor hip width apart. Perform a slight tuck of your pelvis, making your lower back flat and depressing your lower ribs (imagine squashing a grape with your lower back). Focus on holding this posture. Squeeze your glutes to lift your hips up whilst also pressing down with your heels. Stop when you feel like you are unable to control your hips (i.e. if you start wobbling). The height is not important with this exercise, so do not try to go too high. When you can lift your hips up to form a straight line with the rest of your torso in a well-controlled manner. Make sure that your knees stay as wide as your feet. Hold the top position for two to three seconds and repeat 12 times.

2. Marching Bridge with Band

Perform the same two-legged bridge as in the last exercise but pause with your hips in the elevated position. Perform slow alternating kick ups by straightening your leg, as though you were marching. Use a light resistance band around your knees and focus on maintaining the tension on the band throughout the exercise. Make sure your knees stay still and your hips stay level! 20 Repetitions in total

3. One Leg Bridge

To perform a one leg bridge, lie on your back, feet hip width apart with one leg elevated with a 90 degree bend to your hip and knee. The leg will maintain this position during the movement. Perform your bridge pattern but on the single leg. Make sure your hips remain level left to right. Try 10 repetitions on each leg.

One Leg Balance - Targeting Lower Limb (Hip, Knee, Ankle)

Stand with your feet shoulder width apart. Now lift your left foot one inch from the floor. Maintain a straight spinal position as you hold for 15 seconds. Your goal should be to maintain an upright position without leaning to either side. Do 5 repetitions on each foot. You can make this more challenging by balancing on an unstable surface like dense foam or a BOSU ball and by raising your knee to hip height.

Hip Marching - Targeting Hips

Sit on a chair with your feet flat on the floor. Now lift your left knee as high as you can. Lower and repeat on the other leg. Perform 10 repetitions on each leg. To make this exercise slightly harder, resist your upward lift with your hands.

Lunges - Targeting Lower Limb (Hip, Knee, Ankle)

Stand with your feet hip width apart and your hands on your hips. Take a large step forward with your right leg, being sure to maintain an upright torso position but do not lean back. Lower your rear knee down as far as comfortable without it touching the floor. Now push back through the forward thigh to return to your standing start position. Perform 10 repetitions on each leg.

Airplanes - Targeting Core and Lower Limb (Hip, Knee, Ankle)

From a standing position, balance on one leg. Hinge your hips back with the other leg moving behind you. Keep the back leg in line with your torso as it lowers. Place your arms out to the side to balance your body, like wings on a plane. Keep a neutral spine. Hold this position for a few seconds, go back to the starting position and repeat. To make it more challenging try and stay on one leg during the whole set. You can also add a high knee in at the starting position as another modification. This can be a very challenging exercise to start with so by all means hold on to a chair with one arm at first if you need to until you feel more confident. Try 5 repetitions each side at first.

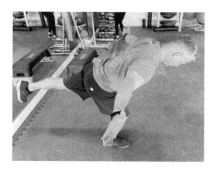

UPPER BODY

Scapulothoracic stability is incredibly important. The scapular stabilizer muscles control your shoulder blades. By coordinating with the rotator cuff (the muscles around your shoulder joint) they control how your arm moves. There are 17 muscles that work around the scapulothoracic joint. Five of the major muscles are:

- The Rhomboids
- Serratus Anterior
- Trapezius
- Levator Scapulae
- Latissimus Dorsi

Weakness in any of these major muscles will affect your shoulder function and how your scapula moves.

As always, there is good news. Here are some great exercises to help aid scapulothoracic stability:

ITYWs

Lie on your tummy face down on the floor keeping your arms to your sides. Make sure your neck is straight. Keep your body still: do not move anything other than your arms and follow these 4 steps by using the letters of the alphabet. *Hold all 4 positions for 10- 15 seconds each or do them dynamically in reps of 10 each.*

1. **I:** Hands down by your sides to create a letter "I", keep palms up and thumbs towards your thighs. Hold position or move them up and down (if doing reps).

2. **T:** Hold your hands out to the sides to create the letter "T" with your arms and body. Hold position or move your arms up and down (if doing reps) with your palms facing ground.

3. **Y:** Now move your arms up in a "Y" position. Hold position or move them up and down (if doing reps) with your palms down.

4. **W:** From the "Y" position, pull your arms into your body leading with the elbows finishing at sides to create a "W." Hold position or move your elbows up and down (if doing reps) squeezing your shoulder blades as you pull down into your body. Repeat sequence 3 times.

Shoulder Blade Squeezes (Scapular Retraction)

Start by relaxing your neck. Stand with feet shoulder width apart and with good posture. Now slowly squeeze your shoulders back and slightly down to avoid shrugging your shoulders. Keep your abdominals and glutes braced. *Hold for 10 - 15 sec before relaxing your shoulders. Repeat 10 - 12 times.*

Band Pull Apart

Stand tall with feet shoulder width apart. Holding a long resistance band with both hands with your palms facing each other and shoulder-width apart. Make sure there is no tension in the band yet. Pull the band apart with both arms to sides as wide as possible, keeping them just below shoulder height squeeze your shoulder blades together and down. Imagine you are trying to stop a tennis ball rolling down your back with your shoulder blades. With tension and control bring your hands back together to starting position. Repeat 12- 15 times.

ADDING STABILITY INTO GYM ROUTINES

As well as these more home based stability exercises, you can also challenge your body by tweaking your everyday resistance exercises at the gym. These could be, weighted single arm and leg exercises or using a Physio (Swiss) or Bosu ball. Here are some examples...

Swiss or Medicine Wall Ball Circles

With your feet shoulder width apart, face a wall holding a Swiss or medicine ball with one arm. Keep the ball shoulder height and press into the wall. Start to roll the ball clockwise making 10 circles. Do the same anti-clockwise and repeat 3 times.

Dumbbell Back Lunges with High Knee

Stand with your feet hip width apart, holding a dumbbell in each hand. Step back into a lunge with your right leg keeping your thigh at the same angle as your torso. Lower your right knee as low as you can go without hitting the ground. Now push back toward the starting position through the left thigh and raising your right knee. Your right knee is now parallel with your hip whilst balancing on your left leg. Hold for 2 seconds, repeat on the same leg for 10 repetitions, then swap legs.

Single Arm Lateral Raise

Stand with your feet hip width apart holding a dumbbell in one hand by your side. Raise your arm out to the side until it's parallel with your shoulder. Hold for 3 seconds. Lower your arm back down for 3 seconds keeping your torso completely still. Repeat 10 times and swap arms.

Single Arm Dumbbell Chest Press

Grab a single dumbbell and lie down on a gym bench. Extend your arm above you so that the dumbbell is over your shoulders but do not lock your elbow joint. Place your other hand on your hip. Slowly bring the dumbbell down to the side of your chest keeping your elbow slightly tucked. Keep your torso still. At the bottom position your elbow should form a right angle to your upper arms. Push back up to bring the dumbbell back to the starting position. Repeat 10 times then swap arms.

Dumbbell Chest Press on a Swiss/ physio ball

Grab a pair of dumbbells and lie down with your upper back on the ball, knees bent with your feet on the ground . Extend your arms above you so that the dumbbells are over your shoulders but do not lock your elbow joints. Slowly bring the dumbbells down to the side of your lower chest. In the bottom position your elbows should form a right angle to your upper arms. Push back up to bring the dumbbells together in the top position. Repeat 12 times.

Squats on a Bosu Ball

Place the blue side of the BOSU ball on the floor. Slowly step onto the flat side, standing with your feet wider than hip-width apart. Slowly push your hips back and bend your knees as you lower down into a squat. Hold for 3 seconds at the bottom. Push through your heels to stand back up to the starting position. Repeat 12 times.

Step Ups with High Knee (alternate legs)

Set up a step to a height that you are able to step onto comfortably. Place one foot on the step and push through your heel to lift your back leg off the ground. Follow through with your back leg raising your knee so it's parallel with your hip and standing tall on the other leg. Step back down and repeat with the other leg. Hold a dumbbell in each hand as a progression. 20 alternating repetitions.

Pallof Press

Fasten a resistance band to a secure anchor point in your gym or at home. Hold the end of the resistance band firmly in both hands. Position yourself away from the anchor point, with the resistance band held at chest height. Keep your feet shoulder-width apart, your knees slightly bent. Keep your feet firmly pushing down into the floor (scrunching your toes helps).Press the resistance band away from your chest, fully extending your arms in front of you without locking your elbows. Hold the resistance band at full extension for 2 - 3 seconds, and slowly release the tension. Return the band to the starting point, and repeat the exercise 12 times. You can also do this as a single arm exercise.

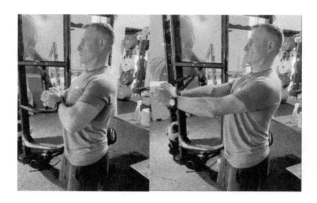

SUMMARY

Improving your stability is perhaps the most important thing you can do to reduce the likelihood that you will become another fall victim. And the great news is, doing so doesn't require a lot of effort. Performing some of these home exercises a couple of times a week can make a huge difference. It can also just take a few minutes - in fact, you can even do them during the ads on TV, or as a quick morning/ before bed routine.

Adding the more gym-based exercises into your routine will also play a huge role in your increased stability and strength.

This is all another piece of the puzzle, but we're now well into our journey of total fitness and there is so much to be optimistic about! Keep focused and your eyes on the prize. Now onto the next stage.

7

AGILITY - NOW THE FUN BEGINS!

AGILITY

I t is the ability to move freely and easily.

Yet, its meaning goes beyond a dictionary definition. An agile person is fit, coordinated, supple, energetic, vibrant and athletic. It's the sort of person that most of us want to be but too few of us actually are.

The benefits of agility training for athletes are well established. It is the most effective way to enhance speed, alertness and coordination. In recent times, there has also been a growing realization of the huge benefits for non-athletes. To appreciate just how agility training can benefit you, let's take a closer look at how our muscles work.

Each of your muscles is made up of connective tissue, muscle tissue, nerves and blood vessels. All of these components coordinate to cause our limbs to move. Each muscle contains thousands of long, thin fibers. These fibers contain two opposing contractile proteins:

- Actin
- Myosin

These proteins repeatedly pull and release against each other. This causes muscular contraction which results in force. When we train the muscle, we enhance its ability to produce this force. This makes us stronger.

Speed, agility and quickness training is governed by what is called the stretch-shortening cycle. The cycle involves a combination of muscle lengthening (eccentric) and muscle shortening (concentric) actions. This acts just like a rubber band that is stretched out and then snaps back. When the eccentric action, such as dropping down into a squat position, comes before a concentric action, such as jumping onto a box, the force output of the concentric action is increased.

Agility training is built around increasing the ability of the stretch-shortening cycle. When you train the stretch-shortening cycle, you increase the connections between the muscles and the brain, allowing you to react faster and to exert more force. As a result, you are able to jump higher, change direction faster and react on the field more quickly.

AGILITY TRAINING BENEFITS

Weight Loss

Agility training is an excellent choice for weight loss. The nature of agility training makes it ideal to be performed in High Intensity Interval Training (HIIT) fashion. This is where you perform all-out effort on an exercise for a short period of time, followed by an even shorter active recovery exercise. You go back and forth between these moves for a set number of rounds.

Here's an example:

> *Stand in front of an agility ladder with a stopwatch in sight. As soon as the timer starts, jump both feet into the first rung of the ladder. Immediately jump them out to the sides of the ladder. Progress up and down the ladder in this manner, moving as fast as you possibly can. When 30 seconds is up, transition to a slow jog up and down the ladder for 10 seconds, before going back to the in-out jump movement for another 30 seconds. Continue until you have completed 8 rounds.*

This type of workout is extremely demanding. Though only taking a few minutes, it will burn a substantial number of calories while you are doing it. It will also bring on the enhanced post-exercise oxygen consumption (EPOC) effect. This will see you burning more calories while you are at rest for up to 38 hours after the workout.

Injury Prevention

Agility training is great for injury prevention. The enhanced balance, control and flexibility that is built as a result of agility training will massively improve your body's ability to maintain proper alignment and coordination when you walk, get up and maneuver your way around. If you stumble, you will be far more able to correct yourself before falling and hurting yourself. This type of training will also improve your posture and body placement, making you less likely to stumble in the first place.

Mind-Body Connection

Agility training, better than any other form of exercise, strengthens the connection between mind and body. As you consistently train yourself in agility movements, they will become second nature and you will develop the ability to move, coordinate, change position and weave without any conscious input.

Balance and Coordination

There is no better form of exercise to enhance your balance and coordination than agility training. By performing quick stop and start, and change of direction agility training exercises, you will be able to move with balanced coordination even when you are engaged in dynamic movement. As a result, your body will work together as a complete unit a lot better. You will also develop the eye-hand and foot coordination required for fast reflexes and reactions.

Better Recovery

Your ability to recover after intense exercise is a critical indicator of your fitness level. Agility training will allow you to build the heart and lung capacity to recover faster.

Faster Results

We've already mentioned how agility training, when done in HIIT fashion, can dramatically speed up your fat loss results. Agility training will actually get you fitter faster across the whole fitness spectrum. The non-linear movement involved with agility training brings into play many of the muscles that are not involved when you perform straight line training.

AGILITY TRAINING APPLIED: PLYOMETRICS

The most effective way to improve your agility is to do some form of plyometric training. Also known as ballistics or jump training, plyometrics involve explosive movement, jumping and quick lateral movement.

When it comes to people over the age of 40, the idea of jumping around may not sound very appealing. After all, their joints and bones are not as limber as they once were. That doesn't mean that they should avoid plyometrics, however. It simply means that you need to approach it smartly.

Smart plyometrics starts with an evaluation of whether you are ready for this form of exercise. A simple test is to take hold of a resistance band and stretch it overhead. From here squat down to full knee bend and then raise straight back up.

If you experience any movement limitation or discomfort while doing this move, you should continue to improve your mobility before you move into plyometric training.

You should also have a base level of strength through your glutes, hamstrings and lower back muscles before you begin plyometric training. You will strengthen these areas through your strength training. I suggest doing at least 12 weeks of strength training to build a foundation of strength in these areas before you introduce plyometrics into your routine.

When you decide that you are ready to incorporate plyometric training into your overall workout plan, I recommend adding them to your routine 1-2 times per week. Because plyometrics involves a lot of effort and requires a strong mind-muscle connection, I do not suggest doing them after your strength training sessions when you are already exhausted from your resistance workout. Performing plyometrics as a stand-alone workout will allow you to give the workout the justice it deserves.

Here is a Plyometric workout that will allow you to improve your agility safely while also increasing your explosive power.

Plyometrics Workout

- Skipping - 2 minutes
- Box Jumps - 60 seconds
- Broad Jumps - 30 seconds
- Skater Jumps - 30 seconds

Skipping

Don't worry if you can't skip - it is a learned practice. Just take it slow and try to build up the number of skips you can do without getting caught up in the rope. Start with skipping on both feet. You can also mimic the exercise without a rope at first to get your endurance up.

Box Jumps

Start with a very low box (less than 12 inches high). Begin with your feet shoulder width apart. Load your body by hinging at the hips, squatting down slightly and swinging your arms back. Now explode up onto the box jumping with both feet lifting at the same time. Land on both feet shoulder width apart into a slight squat and follow through with your arms. Step back down onto the floor and repeat.

Broad Jumps

Begin with your feet shoulder width apart. Load your body by hinging at the hips, squatting down slightly and swinging your arms back. Now jump forward explosively with both feet lifting at the same time. Land on both feet shoulder width apart into a slight squat.

Skater Jumps

Stand with your feet shoulder width apart. Now transfer your weight onto your right leg and lift your left foot off the floor and drop your hips slightly. Now jump to your left by pushing explosively off your right foot. Land on the left leg keeping your knee soft. As soon as you land, reverse the movement to jump back to the right. Try to spend as little time as possible in contact with the floor. Continue this back and forth movement until your time is up.

Agility Ladder Training

After 3 months of doing the above beginner's plyometric training program, you will be ready to add in agility ladder training.

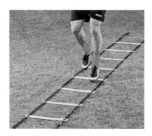

The Agility Ladder is an excellent investment to enhance your agility training. It consists of a rollable ladder made of plastic and canvas that is usually between 10 and 20 ladder rungs long.

Here is a 5 move agility ladder workout...

Agility Ladder Bunny Hops

With both feet together, bunny hop between each rung of your ladder, making light, quick touches in each square with the balls of your feet. When you reach the end rung, swing round and come back again. Imagine that the ground is hot, so that you make the quickest ground contact possible.

Single Leg Hops

Hop down the length of the ladder on one leg, then come back hopping on the other leg. Limit your ground contact to the balls of your feet, moving as quickly as possible. Your goal here is to maintain balance, not touching the rungs of the ladder.

Lateral Bunny Hop

Turn your body side on and bunny hop laterally (sideways) up and down your ladder. It is important to keep your upper body straight up and down on this one. If you lean to the side to build momentum, you will fall at the end.

Icky Shuffle

Start with one foot in the center of the first square and the other out to the side of the ladder. Now step the outside leg into the square, then the other leg out to the other side. Next, move the leg remaining in the rung up to the next square. The sequence is 'one-two-step-up'. Go as fast as you can, without touching your ladder.

Lateral Shuffle

Start with both feet outside the ladder. Step into the ladder with both feet and then out to the other side. As the last foot comes out of the ladder, tap it lightly on the ground and then straight into the next rung. Continue down your ladder. Your verbal cue for this move is 'one-two, one-two, tap and back'.

SUMMARY

Agility is your body's ability to move with grace, control and nimbleness. An agile person is able to adjust and recover, rather than fall and injure themselves. Working on improving your agility will allow you to move better; improve both your balance and recovery time and enhance your mind-body connection. It can also be a lot of fun! However, you need to make sure that your body is ready to take on the increased demands on the muscles and joints that come with agility training. Strength and mobility training will help you to increase your muscle and joint capability to meet these demands.

In the next chapter we will discover yet another foundation that is vital in our total fitness journey. This last physical foundation plays a huge role in every form of exercise we embark on...

8

ENDURANCE - DON'T STOP ME NOW!

NEVER GIVE UP!

It's a three word mantra that fathers pass on to their sons. We cling to it as quality of character, something to be esteemed and aspired to. It is exemplified in words like tenacity and perseverance.

But it all really comes down to endurance.

After all, when we run out of steam, our engine will stop - regardless of how much our mind wills it to keep going!

In this chapter, you are about to discover that the advancing years do not have to sap away at your endurance. In fact, I'm about to show you how you can enhance your get up and go, vitality and endurance every single day.

WHAT IS ENDURANCE?

Endurance is the ability to ward off fatigue for a long period of time. It is the product of a number of factors including:

- Aerobic Capacity
- VO_2 Max
- Lactate Threshold
- Muscle Strength
- Power
- Muscular Endurance

The main limiting factor for endurance is fatigue. Muscular endurance is also dependent on the ratio of fast and slow twitch muscle fibers that your muscles are composed of. Slow twitch muscle fibers have a higher endurance capacity than fast twitch fibers.

Endurance and stamina are often used interchangeably. The subtle difference between them is that endurance is all about the body's physical ability to go on. Stamina also includes mental fortitude.

There are two aspects to endurance:

- Cardiovascular
- Muscular

As we age, our endurance levels will naturally decline. From the age of 45 onwards, we will naturally lose an average of 5 percent of our endurance every decade. The reduction in size of the muscle fibers that occurs with aging results in lower levels of slow twitch muscle fibers. This will negatively impact muscular endurance. Natural loss of muscle function also negatively affects muscular endurance.

As we age, our bodies also become less efficient at using oxygen. Your cardiovascular endurance is dependent upon your body's ability to transport oxygen from the heart to the lungs and then onto the working muscles of the body.

The natural decline in maximal heart rate and VO_2 Max, and the maximum rate of oxygen that your body can use during exercise, also impact on endurance.

The reduced endurance that occurs as we age shows up with increased levels of fatigue. This is shown day to day by walking more slowly, running out of puff after checking the mailbox and having to sit down frequently to 'take a load off'.

Preserving endurance as we age is important for overall health and decreased risk of mortality. One study examined the association between the walking speed of a quarter mile distance and risk of mortality among 3,000 men and women between the ages of 70 and 79. Those with the slowest walking times (which was correlated to lower endurance levels) had the highest risk of death, cardiovascular disease and mobility limitation. 13 percent of the people were unable to complete the quarter mile distance as a result of fatigue.

REVERSING THE ENDURANCE TREND

The good news is that the natural age related endurance decline can be addressed, if not completely reversed. Training to improve your endurance requires that you improve both your cardiovascular and muscular endurance levels.

Improving Cardiovascular Endurance

Exercise to improve your cardiovascular endurance makes you breathe harder, working your heart and lungs and increasing the demand for oxygen. Examples are swimming, brisk walking, jogging, cycling and jumping rope (skipping). However, your cardio endurance program doesn't have to be confined to strict 'exercise' activities. Joining your local tennis/badminton club and playing a game of doubles twice a week or taking up dance lessons are also good options.

FITT-VP

The FITT-VP principle is a useful guideline to base endurance exercise upon. This acronym stands for:

- Frequency
- Intensity
- Time

- Type
- Volume
- Progression

Frequency

Frequency is about the length of each session and the frequency of the activity. If you are new to this type of exercise, start slowly with 10-15 minutes and then work progressively to meet the 150 minutes of cardiovascular exercise per week that is recommended by the American Heart Association. This total will include such other types of cardio exercise as the plyometrics you are doing to improve your agility but not your strength training.

Intensity

Training intensity is a measure of how hard your heart and lungs are working during your endurance workout. The higher the intensity, the greater the endurance-related benefits. Using a heart rate monitor is a good gauge of your aerobic intensity level. Calculate your maximum heart rate by subtracting your age from 220. The following table shows intensity levels as a percentage of maximum heart rate. To calculate your ideal heart rate at each level, multiply your maximum heart rate by the activity factor in the right hand box.

Intensity Level	% age of Max Heart Rate	Activity Factor
Very Light	55%	0.55
Light	60%	0.60
Moderate	70%	0.70
Vigorous	85%	0.85

Time

Time relates to the duration of the workout. Your training time should average about 30 minutes per day.

Type

Type should focus on exercises that involve large muscle groups. When it comes to training modes, cardio activities are grouped into the following four categories:

- Activities that can be done with minimal skill and fitness level (walking, cycling)
- Activities that are more vigorous but don't require a lot of skill (elliptical exercises, jogging)
- Activities that require a certain skill level (swimming, skating)
- Recreational sports (Basketball, tennis)

A well-rounded cardio program will select activities from each of these categories.

Volume

Volume is a measure of the total amount of exercise and is often expressed as total caloric output. Set an initial goal of burning 1,000 calories per week through cardio exercise.

Progression

Progression is the key to making continual improvement in your endurance level. By making your sessions slightly more intense you will be placing an adaptive stress on your cardio system that it will be forced to meet. Start to progress by increasing your training time. Then begin increasing your intensity level.

WARM UP

Spend 5 minutes before your endurance training session warming up. The following routine, which is a combination of dynamic stretching and aerobic warm up, is ideal if you are about to do an activity such as play a team game, ride a bike or go for a jog…

Start with a light jog for 1-2 minutes. If you are about to play a court game, cover the perimeter of the court. This will elevate your heart rate and get you breathing a little heavier.

Once you've got your heart and lungs moving a little, you're ready to lift the intensity slightly with a cardiovascular drill known as 'suicides.' This will lift your heart rate a little more while also stretching out your legs, back and arms. To do this drill, stand on the court sideline or facing a forward area of about 5 meters. Drop down into a sprint start position, with one leg back and the same hand touching the ground. Now jog forward to the centerline (about 2.5 meters), reaching down to touch it with your hand. Pivot and return to the sideline, and touch it with your hands. Now run the entire width of the court (around 5 meters) and touch the opposite sideline. Run back to the other side and again touch the baseline.

Do this forward suicide twice, moving at a jogging pace. Then, do it another two times but this time backpedal on the return each time.

Another great lateral agility warmup is called the Karaoke. This is a side to side shuffle with the added element that you cross one foot over the other with each step. Do this for two lengths of the court. The complexity of this action will engage your mind with your muscles, improving your proprioception and agility.

The aerobic warm up that we've just covered will get your heart rate up and increase your core body temperature in preparation for the game to come. Now you need to do some dynamic stretching in order to warm up your muscles.

Dynamic stretching involves moving your muscles through their full range of motion. Dynamic stretches often simulate the resistance moves that are part of the workout to come, such as doing bodyweight squats or lunges.

DYNAMIC STRETCHING ROUTINE

As well as the dynamic stretches we covered in the Mobility chapter, here is another 6 move dynamic stretching routine that will enhance your mobility ahead of your workout: Bear in mind, you can also mix and match ones from each chapter. It really comes down to how much time you have to warm up.

Hip Rotation x 5

Stand with your feet shoulder width apart. Now lift one leg into the air and rotate from the hip to perform a hip circle in a clockwise direction. After 5 rotations, reverse the motion to perform 5 anti-clockwise hip rotations. Now repeat on the other leg.

You may need to hold onto the tennis net or fence for balance while doing this dynamic stretch.

Knee Circles x 5

Stand with feet shoulder width apart and hands on hips. Now lift one foot slightly off the ground and begin to draw a circle in the air with your knee. The movement will be smaller than in the previous stretch. Perform 5 clockwise followed by 5 anti-clockwise circles. Now repeat on the other leg.

Ankle Circles x 5

Stand with feet shoulder width apart and hands on hips. Now lift one foot slightly off the ground and begin to draw circles with your ankles. This will be the smallest circle yet. Make sure to spread out your toes as you are performing your ankle circles. Again, perform 5 clockwise followed by 5 anti-clockwise circles. Now repeat on the other leg.

Shoulder Shrugs x 10

Stand with your arms extended out to your sides at shoulder level. Now shrug your shoulder blades up and down. This will warm up your shoulder joint and your trapezius muscles. Do this 10 times. Now, maintaining the same arms extended position, hold up your thumbs and then rotate at the wrist, supinate and pronate the hands up and down. Do not bend at the elbows as you do this. Do this 10 times.

SHOULDER CIRCLES

Stand in a neutral position with your arms level with your shoulders, extended away from your body. Keeping your shoulders relaxed, make small circles by rotating your arms backwards five times and then forwards 5 times.

Dynamic Swimmer Stretch x 10

Stand with your arms at your sides. Now bring them across your body to cross over and then extend them back to stretch out your pectoral muscles. In the extension, arch your back to feel the movement through your latissimus dorsi muscles. This action basically involves hugging yourself. Do this for 10 repetitions.

COOLDOWN

Cooling down after exercise or sport play is the most neglected part of being active. You've probably seen this yourself. How many people have you seen who take a few minutes to do some cool down stretches after the game? I'm betting that you could number them on one hand!

You need to be smarter than the majority of people when it comes to prioritizing the cooldown. Those few minutes can make a huge difference to how your body recovers and recuperates from your game or exercise session. A proper cooldown routine will help your muscles, tissues and joints to heal while also promoting enhanced blood flow to fast track nutrients and oxygen to your muscle cells. Once you have completed your main endurance session, you can simply walk for 2-3 minutes around the court, pitch or gym. This will bring your heart rate down gradually to your normal state. This will help to prevent issues like blood pooling, which we will cover later.

The rest of your cooldown will consist of static stretching.

Unlike some of the stretches in the Flexibility chapter that require lying on a mat, here is a sequence of 7 standing stretches that will take just a few minutes to complete...

Arm Stretch

Stand with your arms at your sides and your stomach pulled in, chest expanded and spine in a neutral position (not rounded). Clasp your hands behind your back and slowly lift your arms up, keeping your elbows straight. Hold for 15 - 20 seconds.

Triceps Stretch

Stand in a neutral position with your arms at your sides. Place your left hand behind your back so that your palm sits between your shoulder blades and your elbow points upward. Bring your right hand up behind your back and try to join hands. Hold for 15 - 20 seconds, then repeat with the other arm. You can use a towel to help you until you are able to join your hands.

Quad Stretch

Standing - Hold your foot at the lace part of your shoe (not your ankle), bring it behind your body and tuck your pelvis under so your tailbone is pointing at the wall in front of you (a posterior tilt). Try and get your heel to touch your bum without letting your knee swing out to the side. Hold for 15 - 20 seconds. Repeat with the other leg.

Neck Stretch

With your back straight and your chest lifted, clasp your hands loosely in front of you and relax your shoulders. Keeping your shoulders still, slowly lower your left ear towards your left shoulder. When you have tilted your head as far as is comfortable, hold the stretch. Repeat the stretch to the right.

Repeat this stretch 5 times each side.

Hamstring Stretch

Standing - With your feet hip width apart, place your right leg forward so your right heel is just in front of your left toe. Keeping your right leg straight, place your hands on your left knee and bend the knee. With a straight back, gently lean forward resting your weight on your bent leg. Hold for 15 - 20 seconds.

Overhead Stretch

Stand with your feet hip width apart, your back straight and your head in line with your spine. Lift your arms above your head as far as you can with your palms touching. Do not lean back and arch your lower back. Hold for 15 - 20 seconds. To extend this stretch further, ease your arms back slightly.

Standing Calf Stretch

Stand facing a wall and place your palms on it in line with your chest. Step your right leg back so that it is fully extended with your left knee slightly bent. Now lean forward to the wall, keeping your back foot completely on the floor. You should feel the stretch through your calf muscle. Hold the stretch for 15 - 20 seconds. Repeat on the other leg.

IMPROVING MUSCULAR ENDURANCE

Improving muscular endurance involves increasing the ability of your slow twitch muscle fibers to continue performing for an extended period of time. Very few activities work with your fast twitch or your slow twitch fibers exclusively but there are those which primarily work one of the two. Total fitness requires doing exercises that work both types of muscle fiber.

The following activities will primarily work your slow twitch muscle fibers...Steady state:

- Running
- Swimming
- Cycling
- Brisk Walking

Resistance training, such as the program that is detailed in Chapter 3 of this book, will work both your fast and slow twitch muscle fibers. Because our program includes both high and low rep ranges, you will activate primarily slow twitch fibers with reps higher than 15 and fast twitch fibers with reps below 15.

The current scientific thinking is that it is not possible to increase the number of either your fast or slow twitch muscle fibers. However, you can make them bigger and stronger with consistent training.

The workout protocols that we have already covered, including strength training and your cardiovascular endurance training will also cover your muscular endurance needs. As a result, you do not need to do any separate muscular endurance workouts.

SUMMARY

We have learned that both cardiovascular and muscular endurance are vital to your overall fitness. These types of training can be performed at the gym, at home, out in the park or at your local sports club. As with all exercise, the main ingredient is enjoyment. Take time to find what type of exercise you enjoy and are able to add into your lifestyle.

As we know, starting a new exercise program can be tough and seem daunting at the start, but having come this far in your fitness journey, you have discovered there are so many different components to keeping your body in great shape. Think of yourself like a chef, sprinkling these foundations into your weekly exercise routine. Remember you don't have to go all in right away - instead you should gradually build up all these 6 foundations week to week.

The 6 foundations we have covered so far are all based on physical activity but we still have one of the most important foundations left. This foundation is something that we deal with multiple times a day and can and will make all the difference to how you look and feel...

9

NUTRITION: YOU ARE WHAT YOU (CHOOSE) TO EAT

Y ou are what you eat.

We've heard that statement so often that it has become cliché. But that by no means lessens its importance. You literally are what you eat. Your body is made from the following nutrients contained in food:

- Water
- Protein
- Carbohydrate
- Fat
- Vitamins
- Minerals

Nutrition is the science of how our bodies utilize that food. It boils down to two things:

1. Food's ability to produce energy to allow us to
   function.
2. The nutrients we need to build, maintain and repair
   the organs and systems in our bodies.

As a result, the food that we eat can have a transformative effect on our bodies. When you consistently eat 'unhealthy' foods (e.g. high fat, high salt, processed or sugary foods), your body will suffer. A lack of nutrients can, over time, cause your bones to become brittle, your gums to bleed, and your blood to carry insufficient oxygen to your cells. Too much of certain types of food, such as simple, high glycemic index carbohydrates, will pack unwanted body fat onto your frame. Being overweight or obese brings with it a whole host of related conditions, including cardiovascular disease, diabetes and osteoarthritis. On the other hand, eating foods such as vegetables, fruits, whole grains, beans, nuts and seeds, and lean protein have the benefit of providing the nutrients your body needs to function well without consuming too many calories. The simple fact is that not all foods are created equal. Later in this chapter, we will discuss these foods in more detail.

NUTRITION AND AGING

As we age, our nutritional needs change. Along with the changes such as muscle and bone density loss that we have already identified as affecting us as we grow older, our metabolism slows down and less stomach acid is produced.

Reduced metabolism means that we need to take in fewer calories, but a decrease in stomach acid means that we are less efficient at absorbing the nutrients in the foods we do eat. The micronutrients that have been identified as being difficult to absorb as we age are:

- Vitamin B12
- Calcium
- Iron
- Magnesium

This creates a Catch-22 like dilemma for people in their 40s and beyond; we need to take in *fewer calories* to get *more nutrients* into our bodies. This makes it essential that, if your goal is to achieve good health, body composition and fitness, you need to be more conscious of what you are putting into your mouth with every passing year.

Research has revealed another age related nutritional change - our ability to identify our body's signals for hunger and fullness are decreased. This leads to a decreased appetite as we age that can result in unhealthy weight loss and nutritional deficiencies. Our signals for thirst are also diminished as we age, which could lead to dehydration.

Coupled with the body's natural metabolic decline is the reduced level of activity that is normal with older people. As a result, older people have a lessened need for calories to meet their energy needs. So, if you eat the same amounts of food that you did when you were younger, even if you were eating in a healthy manner, you are likely to pile on unwanted body fat. This extra weight will primarily deposit itself around your belly. This will be more pronounced among post-menopausal women as a result of reduced levels of estrogen.

MACRO & MICRONUTRIENTS

The nutrients in our foods are divided into two categories; Macro (large) and Micro (small). There are technically four macronutrients . . .

- Protein
- Carbohydrate
- Fat
- Alcohol

As alcohol is not essential for life, it is usually not mentioned with the other macros. It contains no minerals, fiber or vitamins, but does supply energy in the form of 7 calories per gram. These are what's known as 'Empty calories'

Micronutrients are the vitamins and minerals that are found in all foods, including herbs and spices. In fact, the micronutrient content of herbs and spices makes it a good idea to flavor your foods with them. This category also includes phytochemicals (found in plant-based foods) and zoochemicals (found in animal-based foods).

Micronutrients are essential to the body because they include the vitamins, minerals and chemical compounds that are vital to a healthy immune system and to the production of energy in the body. Minerals are also important for muscle growth and bone health. Eating a range of different foods will give you a full complement of micronutrients.

THE HEALTHY EATING PLATE

The question of how to get the right balance of macro and micronutrients for optimal health has been written about, debated and studied for decades. It can quickly become confusing for the average person who simply wants to know how they should be eating.

Governments around the world have been providing nutritional guidance to their citizens for decades. The USDA Food Pyramid is the most well-known set of food guidelines on the planet. The pyramid was designed in 1992, with its recommendations being eagerly adopted across the country. The Food Pyramid presented an illustrative representation of six food groups, with their position on a pyramid representing how frequently they should be consumed.

The only problem was that the advice it offered was dead wrong!

The food pyramid was based on the premise that all carbohydrates are good for our health. That is why carb-based foods such as breads and pastas formed the wide base of the pyramid. At the other end of the pyramid, representing its narrow tip, were fats, which were to be consumed sparingly.

As researchers identified the problems with the Food Pyramid, demands were made for an updated version. In 2011, the USDA Food Pyramid was replaced with a colorful plate shaped graphic known as MyPlate to represent the official US Dietary Guidelines. The plate, which is divided into segments to represent food groups, is easier to understand than the confusing food pyramid. MyPlate is divided into four sections:

- Fruits
- Vegetables
- Protein
- Grains

There is also a section, represented by a drinking glass, for water, dairy products and other drinks. Plus a small bottle which represents healthy oils.

Though it was a vast improvement on the Food Pyramid, MyPlate was by no means perfect. Harvard Health Publishing, a division of Harvard Medical School, responded to MyPlate by publishing its own Healthy Eating Plate. It offers more specific and more accurate recommendations for following a healthy diet than MyPlate. In addition, the Healthy Eating Plate is based on the most up-to-date nutrition research, and it is not influenced by the food industry or agriculture policy.

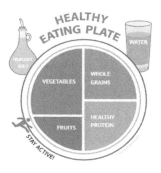

The Harvard Healthy Eating Plate recommends that your plate be made up of . . .

- Fruits and vegetables: ½ plate
- Whole grains: ¼ plate
- Protein: ¼ plate
- Healthy plant oils: in moderation

It also recommends that you drink water, coffee, or tea. You should skip sugary drinks, limit milk and dairy products to a maximum of two servings, and juice to just one small glass per day.

Finally, the figure running around the outside of the Healthy Eating plate is a reminder to stay active.

Let's break down these recommendations further.

VEGETABLES & FRUITS

Vegetables should form the basis of your diet. They are the most nutrient dense foods that exist, containing the vitamins, minerals and phytochemicals that your body needs to work at its best. Eating a variety of types and colors of vegetables and fruits provides your body with the mix of nutrients that it needs.

Here are some tips to help you increase your vegetable and fruit intake:

- Place fruit where you can see it - in a bowl on the kitchen counter or chopped up, fruit salad style in a bowl in the fridge.
- Go exploring down the produce aisle and regularly try new vegetables.
- Aim to get at least one serving each of the following daily; dark green leafy vegetables, red fruits & vegetables, legumes & peas, citrus fruits.

WHOLE GRAINS

Always choose whole grains over refined grains, which have been stripped of valuable nutrients during processing. There are three parts to the whole grain kernel:

- Bran
- Germ
- Endosperm

The bran is packed with fiber and contains the B-Vitamins, iron, copper, zinc, magnesium, antioxidants and phytochemicals. The germ is the core of the kernel and is a rich source of healthy fats, Vitamin E, B Vitamins, antioxidants and phytochemicals. The endosperm is the interior part of the kernel that contains the carbohydrate and protein.

Fiber is essential to healthy digestion and weight control. It slows down the breakdown of carbohydrates into glucose. This helps to balance out blood sugar levels and prevent sharp spikes in insulin release. Fiber also reduces unhealthy LDL cholesterol level and improves the movement of waste through the intestinal tract.

Emphasizing increased fiber intake over the age of 50 will help you to offset such issues as irregular bowel movements and digestive system upset. Having said this, it is important that your fiber intake is also high at a younger age. I myself have suffered from diverticulitis (an infection or inflammation of the intestines) in my early 30s. This was partly brought on by (amongst other factors) a fiber intake below the recommended levels.

You need to be careful when buying whole grains as some foods that are labeled as whole grain are not what they seem. The USDA provides the following 5 criteria for selecting healthy whole grains:

1. Whole grain' is the first ingredient on the ingredients list
2. Added sugars are not one of the first three ingredients
3. The word "whole" is included before any grain ingredient
4. A carbohydrate-to-fiber ratio of less than 10:1
5. The industry-sponsored Whole Grain Stamp

PROTEIN

Protein is the building material which the body uses to construct every part of you. There are more than 10,000 types of proteins in your body, and they are all made up of chains of amino acids. There are twenty amino acids, and nearly half of these (to be specific, nine) cannot be made by the body. These are called the essential amino acids and must be obtained from the foods we eat.

The UDS National Academy of Medicine recommends that adults consume a minimum of 0.8 grams of protein for every kilogram of body weight. However, for more active individuals this number needs to increase. The American college of sports medicine recommends a protein intake of 1.2 - 1.7 grams of protein per kilogram. In contrast, the International society of sports nutrition recommends 1.4 - 2 grams per kilogram. If we take both recommendations into account, we can come to a daily range of 1.2 -2 grams of protein for every kilogram of body weight.

This can understandably get confusing but it really comes down to what kind of exercise you're doing. Resistance based training - particularly activities like bodybuilding - will be at the higher end of 1.6 - 2 grams per Kilogram. On the other hand, more endurance -based exercises such as running or cycling would be at the lower end of 1.2-1.6 grams per Kilogram

The healthiest protein sources are fish, poultry, beans, nuts, red meat and cheese.

WATER

For millions of years, water was the only fluid that humans consumed. Our ancient ancestors only began drinking milk when animals were domesticated. Then followed the introduction of beer and wine. Today the amount of fluid choices is mind boggling, with the result that water, considered by many to be plain, tasteless and boring, is consumed far less frequently than it should be.

Your body thrives on water. In fact, every cell in your body soaks it up. 60% of your body weight is composed of water. To put that another way, if you're a 140-pound woman, 84 of those pounds are water!

The precise amount of water that you are carrying depends upon your body composition. Here's the water content of four major body constituents:

- Bone – 22%
- Fat Tissue – 25%
- Muscle – 75%
- Blood – 83%

We can divide the water in the body into two categories:

- Intracellular Fluid (ICF)
- Extracellular Fluid (ECF)

Around two thirds of the water in your body is intracellular, which means that it is contained within the cells. It contains a large amount of potassium and magnesium and a small amount of sodium and chloride. The rest of the water inside your body is found outside of the cell membranes. Of that amount, a quarter is contained within the vascular system, and makes up the plasma component of blood volume. The other three quarters is known as interstitial fluid, which is the fluid solution that surrounds your cells and connective tissue.

Without the right amount of water, your body will not function properly. Just take a look at what water does for you every second, without your realizing it:

- Regulates body temperature
- Lubricates joints
- Moistens tissues for mouth, eyes and nose
- Protects body organs and tissues
- Helps prevent constipation
- Helps dissolve minerals and other nutrients to make them accessible to the body
- Helps convert food to energy
- Carries nutrients and oxygen to the cells

Not only does it do all this, but the brain is composed of almost 75% water. Keeping the brain saturated prevents memory loss associated with aging. Drinking more water helps your kidneys and liver flush toxins out of your body. This will make your skin clearer and more radiant. Dehydration reduces the amount of blood in the body, forcing the heart to pump harder in order to deliver oxygen-bearing cells into our muscles.

Still not convinced how vital water is to your life? Then consider this:

You will still survive if you lose 50% of your body's glucose (energy), fat or protein.

You will die if you lose more than 20% of your body's water!

HOW MUCH WATER DO YOU NEED?

You may have heard the recommendation to drink 8 glasses of water each day. This is a good general guideline but may not be appropriate for everybody. The US National Academy of Medicine recommends a daily water intake of 13 cups for men and 9 cups for women. 1 cup is equivalent to 250 ml (9 oz).

Higher amounts will be needed by people who exercise or are involved in activities that cause them to sweat. The workout programs outlined in this book require that you increase your water intake. We recommend that you carry a water bottle with you throughout your workout and sip from it liberally.

You can determine whether your water intake is appropriate by looking at the color of your urine. Ideally, your urine should be straw colored, indicating that you are well hydrated. The darker your urine is, the less water you have in your body. So, if your urine is amber or honey colored, take this as a sign that you need to drink more water.

ELECTROLYTES

When we talk about electrolytes, we are referring to minerals that have the job of, among other things, facilitating the passage of fluids through cell membranes. Five key electrolytes are:

- Magnesium
- Sodium
- Potassium
- Chloride
- Calcium

Electrolytes also help to maintain a healthy pH level. This is a measure of how acidic or alkaline the body's solution is. When our electrolytes are out of balance, the body's fluids will tend to be overly acidic, which can cause a whole host of health problems.

It is vital to healthy body functioning that we have a proper balance of electrolytes. As with fluid intake, this balance depends upon the difference between electrolyte intake and electrolyte loss.

We lose electrolytes through urine and sweat. In order to replace them following intense exercise, researchers suggest taking a carbohydrate drink that is infused with electrolytes during and after the session.

You can help to maintain a healthy electrolyte balance by eating foods that are rich in electrolyte minerals. Here are five to get you started:

- Cheese (for sodium)
- Bananas (for potassium)
- Table salt (for chloride)
- Walnuts (for magnesium)
- Milk (for calcium)

CALORIC INTAKE

The fundamental reason that we eat is to supply the energy that our bodies need to function. If we don't supply enough of it through food, the body will draw upon its reserve energy source (stored body fat) to provide it. If we consume more than we need, the excess is stored on the body as reserve energy. Getting the right balance between energy intake and energy expenditure will largely determine whether we lose, gain, or maintain weight.

Energy from food is measured in calories. It is the amount of heat required to raise one liter of water one degree Celsius. When calories are consumed, they release heat, which is the energy that fuels us.

In the 19th century, a system was designed to affix a caloric amount to food. So, when we say that a food contains a certain number of calories, we have an indication of how much energy it will provide for the body. We are also able to determine the level of activity required to burn up calories. From this we can determine the caloric payoff for different types of exercise as well as the approximate number of calories the body requires each day to function.

A simplistic way to think about calories is in terms of a bank account. Your account is the store of calories in your body. Deposits are the calories you consume. Withdrawals are the calories you use up each day. If, at the end of the day, you have a surplus in your account, the number of stored calories will increase and you will gain weight. If you have a deficit, you will lose weight.

The reality is that it is more complicated than that. All calories are not created equal, the rate the body burns calories for energy is constantly changing, and the cascade of hormones throughout your body also play their part. However, the law of energy balance gives us a good ballpark figure to how many calories we need to consume each day.

In order to work out your daily caloric requirement, you first need to know how many calories your body uses up each day.

Basal Metabolic Rate (BMR)

Your BMR is the number of calories that your body needs to sustain all of your body's functions while you are at rest. It accounts for 65 percent of your total caloric consumption. The other 35 percent comes from activity. About 80 percent of BMR is determined by lean body mass. The more muscle you have on your body, the higher your BMR will be. That is why one of the best things you can do to lose fat is to build muscle!

Working Out Your BMR

There are several ways to work out your BMR. One of the easiest and most reliable is what is known as the **Harris-Benedict Equation**. Although effective, this equation was updated in 1990 by Mifflin and St Jeor with around a 5% higher accuracy level. You could use either equation, but below I've used the more accurate **Mifflin and St Jeor** calculation.

An important fact to note before you begin is that this equation only works with metric units. If you know your weight in pounds and height in feet, you will need to convert these to kg and cm, respectively, before you begin.

Men:

BMR (kcal/day) = (10 x weight (kg)) + (6.25 x height (cm)) - (5 x age (years)) + 5

Women:

BMR (kcal/day) = (10 x weight (kg)) + (6.25 x height (cm)) - (5 x age (years)) - 161

Let's run through the equation with the example of a 70kg woman who is 60 years of age and 167 cm tall. Note, it's important to keep the brackets in, otherwise you will end up with a squiffy result!

$$\text{BMR} = (10 \times 70) + (6.25 \times 167) - (5 \times 60) - 161$$
$$= \textbf{1283 calories per day}$$

This tells us that this woman needs to take in 1283 calories each day just to stay alive. But that doesn't account for any physical activity. To work out what out her caloric maintenance level is, we need to multiply the BMR by an activity factor as follows:

Exercise Level	Activity Factor
No Exercise	1.2
Exercise 1-3 times per week	1.375
Exercise 4-5 times per week	1.55
Exercise 6-7 times per week	1.725
Very labor-intensive job	1.9

Our 60-year-old woman exercises 1-3 times per week. So her activity factor is 1.375.

We need to multiply her BMR by that activity factor:

1283 x 1.375 = 1764 calories per day

Now is the time to do these calculations for yourself to know exactly how many calories need to be put into your body to maintain your current body weight. Once you know that number, then you will be able to adjust to burn body fat every single day.

Use the appropriate formula above to work out your BMR.

My BMR = _____calories

Now multiply that figure by your selected Activity Factor to get your Caloric Maintenance Level.

My Caloric Maintenance Level = _____calories

This is the number of calories you need to consume per day to maintain your weight. If you want to change your weight, there is one final step...

To lose body fat, subtract 500 calories per day.

To add lean muscle, add 500 calories per day.

Now we know about our ideal caloric intake and how to build a healthy and varied food plate, let's take a look at how you could apply this in your daily life.

SAMPLE DAILY MENU

Before Breakfast (½ liter water)

Breakfast

Cinnamon Apricot Breakfast Couscous

---

3 CUPS SKIM MILK, ONE 2-INCH CINNAMON STICK, 1 CUP DRY WHOLE-WHEAT COUSCOUS, ½ CUP DRIED APRICOTS, CHOPPED ¼ CUP RAISINS, 5 TEASPOONS BROWN SUGAR, PINCH OF SALT, 4 TEASPOONS CANOLA OIL

1. Pour the milk into a medium saucepan and drop in the cinnamon stick. Heat the milk over medium-high heat until small bubbles form around the edges. 2. Remove the saucepan from heat and stir in the remaining ingredients, reserving 1 teaspoon of brown sugar. 3. Cover and let the couscous stand for 10 to 15 minutes, or until the couscous absorbs the liquid. Remove and discard the cinnamon stick. 4. Sprinkle the remaining teaspoon of brown sugar on top to serve.

OR Poached Egg on Toast with Avocado Mash

---

2 MEDIUM POACHED EGGS, ½ AN AVOCADO MASH, 1 SLICE WHOLEMEAL TOAST, 5 CHERRY TOMATOES, HANDFUL OF SPINACH, WATERCRESS AND ARAGULA MIXED SALAD, TABLESPOON EXTRA VIRGIN OLIVE OIL, SQUEEZE OF LEMON JUICE

1. Boil the water with a squeeze of white wine vinegar for the eggs, mash the avocado into a bowl, cut the cherry tomatoes in half. 2. Put the toast on and poach the 2 eggs for 2- 2 ½ minutes on a medium heat. 3. When the toast is done, spread the avocado on the toast and place the tomatoes on top. 4. When the eggs are done place them on some kitchen towel to soak up the water. 5. Add the salad on the plate and drizzle with lemon and extra virgin olive oil, take the eggs off the towel and place on the plate, season with salt and pepper.

Snack

Apple + handful of walnuts or almonds

Lunch

Tuna salad with capers & olives

10–12 OUNCES CANNED TUNA (1–2 CANS) IN WATER, DRAINED ¼ CUP DICED CELERY, 3 TABLESPOONS FRESH LEMON JUICE, 2 TABLESPOONS CHOPPED ALMONDS, 2 TABLESPOONS RINSED AND CHOPPED CAPERS, 1 TABLESPOON EXTRA-VIRGIN OLIVE OIL, 1 TABLESPOON CHOPPED FRESH DILL SALT AND FRESHLY GROUND PEPPER

1. Flake the tuna with a fork into a mixing bowl. 2. Add the remaining ingredients except the salt and pepper, and stir until well combined. Season with salt and pepper. 3. Serve on wholemeal toast and/or a bed of greens.

Snack

2 tablespoons hummus with 8 baby carrots

Dinner

Italian Herbed Lamb Chops

2 TABLESPOONS EXTRA-VIRGIN OLIVE OIL, 1 TABLESPOON MINCED GARLIC, 6 BONE-IN LAMB CHOPS 1½ INCHES THICK, SALT AND FRESHLY GROUND PEPPER, 2 TABLESPOONS WHOLE-WHEAT FLOUR, 2 TABLESPOONS PLAIN BREAD CRUMBS, 1 TEASPOON DRIED OREGANO, ¼ TEASPOON DRIED THYME, ½ TEASPOON DRIED ROSEMARY

1. Heat the olive oil and garlic in a heavy skillet over medium-low heat. 2. Season the lamb chops with salt and pepper. 3. Combine the flour, bread crumbs, and herbs in a shallow dish and dredge the lamb chops to coat. 4. Arrange the chops in the skillet and cook for 5 to 7 minutes on each side, or until lightly browned, flipping every 3 minutes. 5. Let the chops rest in the skillet for 3 to 4 minutes before serving. Serve with your choice of green or red vegetables, legumes & peas, sweet potato mash.

Dessert

Simple Lemon Sorbet

---

1 CUP WATER, ¾ CUP SUGAR, ¾ CUP FRESH LEMON JUICE

1. Whisk together the water and sugar in a saucepan over medium heat. Stir until the sugar dissolves. Remove the sugar water from the heat and set aside. 2. Whisk in the lemon juice, then cover the mixture and chill it until cold. 3. Pour the mixture into a shallow pan and freeze it for 1 hour. Stir the mixture, then refreeze it until it is solid. 4. Just before serving, break the sorbet into pieces and blend it smooth in a food processor.

OR Easy Greek Yogurt

150g GREEK YOGURT, HANDFUL MIXED BERRIES, SPRINKLE OF MIXED SEEDS AND WALNUTS, DRIZZLE OF HONEY

1. Scoop the yogurt into the bowl. 2. Add the berries, walnuts and seeds on top. 3. Drizzle the honey...easy!

SUMMARY

As we have discovered in this chapter, nutrition is just as important - if not more so - than my other 6 foundations of total fitness. Consider that we eat 3-5 times a day, and there is temptation everywhere! Every few hours, we have to make decisions that can affect the way we look and feel. Luckily, we can use the simple Healthy Eating Plate to keep us on track. We now know about the key macro and micronutrients that are essential to keep us fit and healthy, and how we may need to adapt our nutrition to account for our changing metabolism as we grow older.

Digging deeper into nutrition requires another book in itself but when it all comes down to it, the vast majority of us do have the ability to change the way we eat for the better with willpower, controlled portions and a consistent routine. The good news is, life is all about balance so do enjoy treating yourself in moderation - and when you do, make sure you enjoy it!

We've been on a real journey together over the course of this book! We have now covered all 7 of my foundations of total fitness, and you should be feeling confident and motivated to get started with your new lifestyle. The best version of you is yet to come! Our final chapter will walk us through warming up and cooling down - vital for our preparation for, and recovery from, exercise.

10

WARM UP, COOLDOWN AND RECOVERY

WARMING UP & COOLING DOWN

Warming up and cooling down before and after an exercise session is something that we all know we should be doing. Yet, very few people give it the time and attention that it deserves. Many don't warm up at all, simply throwing themselves into the thick of their workout. You might be able to get away with that sort of recklessness in your teens or your 20s, but certainly not in your 40s or beyond.

Unless you ingrain the habit of gradually increasing your body's readiness for exercise you will suffer the consequences. Just think of what happens when you go to start your car on a cold, frosty morning. Don't you let it warm up for a minute or two before you take it out onto the highway? Doing so will allow its engine to run more efficiently. You, too, will operate more efficiently when you warm up before exercise.

When you are in a non-exercise state, around 20 percent of your body's total blood volume is contained in the muscles, with the balance being in our organs. When you warm up, you are able to transfer more blood from your organs to your muscles. That blood brings oxygen and nutrients into your working muscle cells. The blood then carries waste products out of the muscle cell.

The gradual increase of movement that occurs when you warm up also warms up your joints and lubricates them so they are primed for exercise movement.

Your warm up should feel quite easy. It is designed to get your body ready for the more intense work to follow. In a couple of chapters, we have already included specific warm up and cooldown routines that will gently prepare you for the workout and then return you to a state of inactivity.

It is important to also warm up thoroughly before you engage in any sport or active game activity. Whether you are playing pickleball or going for a jog through the park, it is vital that you ease your body into the activity. The one time that you skip your warmup because you're late or your team-mates are ready to get started is the one time that you will suffer an injury!

Cooling down is just as important. After intense resistance training or cardiovascular endurance like a long run or sprint session, your body is in a state of raised alert and it needs a small amount of time to gradually come back down to the safe zone. Think of it like driving a car at 70mph and all of a sudden slamming on the brakes! As you can imagine, this wouldn't be good for the car - or anything inside it.

When you are in a state of raised alert following exercise, your heart rate and breathing are both high as well as your blood pressure. A gradual return to your resting heart rate will help avoid dizziness or fainting. Feeling nauseous, dizzy or faint after exercise is usually caused by what is known as venous (blood) pooling. Blood is diverted to your muscles during exercise to ensure they have adequate oxygen to sustain the contractions required. This muscular contraction effectively squeezes your veins, which helps them to return your blood back to your heart against the pull of gravity. Venous pooling refers to the buildup of blood in your veins after the muscles in your limbs stop contracting following intense exercise, and normally occurs if you have not cooled down properly. Just a few minutes of rhythmic muscle contraction will be enough to help your blood return to your heart. Your blood pressure dropping will also assist the transition for blood from the lower extremities to return to resting flow patterns. This can all sound a bit scientific so here are a few easy things you can do to cool down:

1. Walk around the room or on a treadmill for 3-5 minutes.

2. Perform static stretches and if you have extra time, light foam rolling.

3. Focus on relaxing and breathing during the cool down. Remember you are winding down to go back to your day.

RECOVERY

Ensuring that you are fully recovered between exercise sessions is key to ensuring that you perform at your best and reduce your chance of injury. As they age, many people notice that their ability to recover is impaired significantly. In this section, we identify three things you can do to ensure that you maximize your recovery.

Sleep

Most people don't factor sleep into the recovery process. In fact, it is arguably the most important factor of them all. It is during this time that your muscles recover, repair and rebuild the muscle tissue that has been broken down during your workout. To achieve this, it needs around 8 hours of deep, restful slumber.

Obviously, when your body is resting through the night, it isn't being called upon to carry out all of the energy demanding requirements of the day. This allows it to concentrate on recovery and repair.

It is also during the hours that you are lying in your bed that a pair of extremely powerful hormones are released to do their work. These two hormones are . . .

- Human Growth Hormone
- Testosterone

As you probably already know, these two hormones are essential for muscle recovery, repair and growth.

Interrupted sleep is a key sign of overtraining, so it is important to monitor your sleep. If your sports watch or fitness tracker has a sleep monitoring function on it, be sure to make use of it. If you do create an overnight sleep debt prior to your workout, try to get a power nap after your training session. Even twenty minutes will be sufficient to make up the lost sleep.

For many active people it is a challenge to come to terms with sleep. They tend to view it as a sign of laziness. However, in order to optimize your training and recovery, you need to get out of that mindset and start to view sleep as an integral part of a smart training program.

Here are 7 hacks to ensure that your sleep is of the highest quality...

- Plan to get to bed at the same time every night and to wake up at the same time in the morning. I can't overstate the importance of routine!

- Maintain a dark, cool and quiet bedroom environment.
- Keep all forms of entertainment, including TVs, computers and tablets out of your bedroom.
- Avoid being active within 2-3 hours of bedtime. Spend that time winding down, both physically and mentally. An hour before retiring, turn off the TV, do your daily journaling and read a book.
- Don't consume caffeine after 2pm.
- Have a warm bath or shower about 90 minutes before bed. The hot water helps to lower your body temperature, which helps signal to the body that it's time for bed.
- Have a cup of herbal tea or hot milk an hour before going to bed.

Hydration

After reading Chapter Nine, you already know how important it is to drink water between workouts and while you are exercising. It's essential to replace lost body fluids and keep up your energy and strength levels.

But you shouldn't stop there. It is just as important to drink plenty of water AFTER your session has finished. After the workout your body is in a state of stress. Taking in a constant supply of water will lubricate it and help everything to work more efficiently. It will also allow the nutrients that your body needs straight after the workout (fast acting carbohydrates and protein) to get to the cells much faster.

Nutrition

In the previous chapter, we discussed the importance of a balanced diet for total fitness. I also outlined a suggested plan to hit your nutrition goals as outlined by the Healthy Eating Plate. However, if you are working out on a given day, you also need to consider the timing of your meals. About 90 minutes beforehand (120 minutes if you are swimming) you should have a whole food meal. This time window will give your body plenty of time for digestion before the added stress of your workout kicks into play. By the time you start your exercise, the nutrients will be coursing through your bloodstream in order to provide the fuel you need to move your muscles.

That pre-workout meal needs to contain a lean protein source and some slow release carbohydrates. Choose an easily digestible lean protein such as fish rather than red meat. The slow release carbs will give your muscles a constant energy supply over the next couple of hours. A great choice would be a large baked sweet potato, a palm sized chicken breast and broccoli.

Your workout will deplete the glycogen stores in your liver. Replace it by having a couple of bananas in the hour or so after your session.

CONCLUSION

In the introduction to this book, I made the rather bold claim that getting weaker, less conditioned and feebler as you age doesn't have to be your future lot in life. I told you that you don't have to conform to society's template of aging; that you could, in fact, become fitter, healthier and more agile with each passing year. In our journey from there to here, we have plotted our way through the roadmap to achieve those outcomes. This final chapter brings all of that information together to show you exactly how to implement it into your life.

So, let's recap and summarize our journey together. We began by taking an eyes wide open look at what happens to our bodies when we age. We discovered that our hearts become less efficient at pumping blood around our body, our bones become less dense, our muscles get smaller and weaker, our key hormones change in their output levels, our sleeping patterns change, our metabolism slows down, and we become fatter!

But...and this is the crucial point – we also learned that, though we may not be able to reverse all of the effects of aging, we can most definitely slow them down.

The key to thriving, rather than just surviving, as we age is summed up in the single word 'fitness'. We found out, however, that fitness is a far more holistic, encompassing concept than most people consider it to be. In fact, total fitness incorporates the following 7 foundations, that we can consider like the foundations of a building...

- Strength
- Flexibility
- Mobility
- Stability
- Agility
- Endurance
- Nutrition

We then began drilling down on each of those 7 foundations.

Strength training, we discovered, is a key to reversing the effects of aging. At that point, I made another bold statement (you may be starting to see a trend here). That statement bears repeating...

No matter your age or ability now, you NEED to take up strength training and perform it consistently over the course of the rest of your life. It is never too late to start and, as soon as you do, your body and your mind will start to reap immediate benefits.

You were then provided with a basic sample strength training program that divided your body into two halves (upper and lower/core), so that you were working your upper body one day and your lower body and core the next.

We then introduced the aspect of mobility and provided you with a 3-part mobility drill to incorporate into your strength training warm-up. It comprised:

- Myofascial tissue massage to release and loosen muscles
- Dynamic stretching
- Mobility drills

Static stretching was brought in as a key component of your post-strength workout cooldown. This will, not only make you become more flexible, but will also help avoid injures and muscle soreness in the coming hours and days post workout.

We learned that stability exercises are a vital component in helping to prevent falls and avoid imbalances. We learned that the two aspects of stability that we need to train are active stability and passive stability, and looked at strategies to achieve these. We also looked at specific exercises to improve the stability of the core, lower limbs, lumbar spine, and shoulders.

When it comes to the next important fitness foundation - agility - we identified plyometric training as an ideal way to enhance that aspect of fitness. A four move plyometric workout was provided, with a more advanced agility ladder sequence as an agility training progression.

Endurance training, the sixth foundation of total fitness, involves two aspects: cardio and muscular endurance. Increasing your cardiovascular endurance can be achieved with swimming, brisk walking, jogging, cycling, and rope jumping. Playing active games you enjoy with your friends and family are also great ways to improve your cardio endurance. To enhance your muscular endurance, you should perform high repetitions on your strength workouts, in the 15 plus rep range. These have already been built into your strength training program.

The final foundation of total fitness that we discussed was nutrition. We identified the Harvard Healthy Eating Plate Model as a healthy, complete and balanced model to follow.

The Healthy Eating Plate promotes:

- A wide variety of vegetables and fruits
- A variety of whole grains
- Limited refined grains

- Healthy lean protein options like fish, poultry, beans and nuts
- Healthy oils, such as olive and canola oil for cooking, and on salads
- Plenty of water, supplemented by coffee and/ or a glass or two of milk daily

Let's now bring each of the 6 movement aspects of total fitness together into a weekly plan. Remember that your mobility drill and flexibility work bookend your strength training as the warm up and cooldown routines. You can however also add mobility drills into your main workout, as they can be done in between your resistance sets while you recover. It can get boring just waiting for the next set of weights and watching the clock tick, so doing a set of Cat Cows or Fire Hydrants in between your squats or bench press exercises can be very time efficient.

Below are two different example weekly routines that incorporate all 6 aspects in slightly different ways.

Weekly Total Fitness Plan 1

Mon	Tues	Wed	Thurs	Fri	Sat	Sun
Mobility Drills	*Mobility Drills*	Agility Training	*Mobility Drills*	*Mobility Drills*	Cardio Endurance	**Rest**
Strength Upper Body	**Strength Lower Body**	Stability Drills	**Strength Upper Body**	**Strength Lower Body**		
Plus: 5-10 mins Static Stretching	*Plus:* 5-10 mins Static Stretching	*Plus:* 5-10 mins Static Stretching	*Plus:* 5-10 mins Static Stretching	*Plus:* 5-10 mins Static Stretching	*Plus:* 5-10 mins Static Stretching	

Weekly Total Fitness Plan 2

Mon	Tues	Wed	Thurs	Fri	Sat	Sun
Full Body Resistance Exercise & Mobility Drills	Stability Drills & Corrective Exercises	Full Body Resistance Exercise & Mobility Drills	Agility Drills & Corrective Exercises	Full Body Resistance Exercise & Mobility Drills	Cardio Endurance	Rest
Plus: 5-10 mins Static Stretching	*Plus:* 5-10 mins Static Stretching	*Plus:* 5-10 mins Static Stretching	*Plus:* 5-10 mins Static Stretching	*Plus:* 5-10 mins Static Stretching	*Plus:* 5-10 mins Static Stretching	
	Optional Cardio: Brisk Walk- 30 mins **or** Steady Jog- 20 mins		*Optional Cardio:* Brisk Walk- 30 mins **or** Steady Jog-20 mins			

We've now come to the end of the book, but this is just the beginning of your journey. All that remains now is to put what you have learned into practice. We all have different weekly routines and work schedules, so my advice is to incorporate these 7 foundations in a routine that you are able to be consistent with, alongside a healthy eating regime.

And that is perhaps the greatest challenge of them all.

You see, the majority of people who purchase fitness books get to this stage, end up with a head full of potentially life changing knowledge and then do...

...Nothing!

Procrastination and familiarity lead them back to their old way of doing things - you know, the very pattern of eating and non-activity that led them to buy the book in the first place.

So, the question before you now is this...

Are you going to revert back to the old, familiar, but body diminishing ways of old?

OR

Are you going to accept the challenges that have been presented before you, embrace the workout challenge and start thriving as the years advance, turning back the ravages of time and giving your body the respect it deserves?

...the choice is yours.

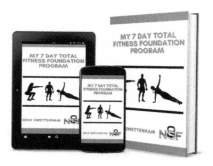

A Special Gift For My Readers

Included with the purchase of this book is My 7 Day Total
Fitness Foundation Program to help you get started on your
fitness journey. This program is a great way to start or adapt
your training using all my 7 foundations.
Click the link below and let us know which email address you
would like it delivered to.

www.nickswettenhamfitness.com

Decline Dumbbell Press

Set an exercise bench to a 30 degree decline. Grab a pair of dumbbells and lie down on the bench. Extend your arms above you so that the dumbbells are over your lower chest. Slowly bring the dumbbells down to your torso. In the bottom position your elbows should form a 90 degree angle to your upper arms. Push back up to bring the dumbbells together in the top position.

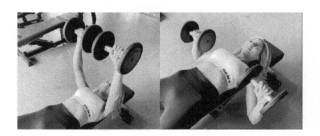

One Arm Lat Pull In

Place a seat in front of a cable pulley machine. Set the pulley on the highest setting and position the bench a few feet in front of the machine. Now sit side on to the machine and reach up to grab the cable with your closest arm. Adjust your position until your arm is at a 30 degree angle.

From this starting position, pull in and down until your elbow is down to hip height. Focus on fully contracting and extending your lats throughout the movement. See picture in chapter 3.

Shrugs

Hold a pair of dumbbells at arm's length with your palms facing into your thighs. Now, without bending the elbows, shrug your shoulders up and back in a circular motion.

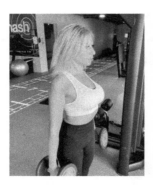

Cable Side Lateral Raises

Set the pulley on a cable pulley machine at hip height. Stand side on to the machine and grab the cable in your outside arm. With a straight arm bring the cable out and up to shoulder level. Slowly lower and return. See picture in chapter 3.

Cable Front Deltoid Press

Place a seat with a 90 degree upright a few feet in front on a double cable pulley machine, facing away from it. Set the pulley at hip height (when seated on the bench). Grab the handles and sit on the bench. Start with your hands by your sides with your elbows slightly behind your torso, palms up. Now push your arms forward and up to full extension in front of your body but do not lock your elbows. See picture in chapter 3.

Rear delt cable extension

Stand facing a cable pulley machine and about 3 feet away from it with the pulley set to eye height. Hold each handle but with the opposite hand so your arms cross over. Pull your arms out to the side then back behind your body squeezing your shoulder blades together. Slowly bring back to start position. See picture in chapter 3.

Cable Torso Rotation

Stand side on to a cable pulley machine and about three feet away from it with the pulley set at hip height. Grab the handle in both hands with arms extended in front of your body. Now rotate from the hips to twist away from the pulley machine. Return and repeat.

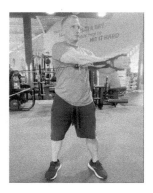

Cable Crunch

Place a seat with a back support about three feet in front of a cable pulley machine and facing away from it. Set the pulley to its highest setting. Place a rope handle on the cable. Now grab the handle with both hands and sit on the seat. The rope handles will now be at the side of your head. Crunch down to full contraction and then back to full extension.

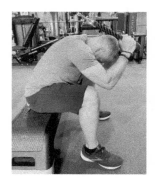

Seated Torso Extension

Sit on a seat with a light dumbbell held against your chest. Now round your spine forward to full contraction and then arch back to fully extend the lower back muscles. This is the same movement as the cable crunch but the resistance is operating in the other direction.

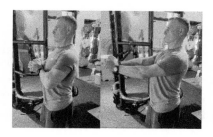

Cable Squat

Set the cables on a double pulley machine to the lowest setting. Face the machine and grab the handles stepping back a few steps. Try to stay upright as you squat down to a full squat. The weight should prevent you from falling back. Push through the heels to return to the start position. See picture in chapter 3.

Goblet Squat

If you are using a dumbbell, hold it vertically. Stand with feet shoulder width apart. Leading with your hips, lower your body into a squat keeping your feet flat on the ground. Keep your elbows inside your knees and go as low as you can maintaining a neutral spine (straight back and neck) Push through with your heels and stand tall without leaning back.

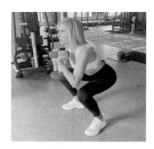

Glute kickback machine

Position your forearms on the machine pads and grip the handles. Maintain an engaged core and neutral spine. Place the arch of your foot onto the footpad and make sure your knee is in line with your hip. In a smooth motion, kick back to extend your hip and knee then squeeze your glute. Do not lock out your knee. Reverse the motion slowly with control.

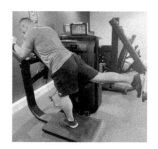

Seated Leg Curl

Position yourself on the seated leg curl machine at your local gym. Keep your hips, knees and toes in line. Pull down on the leg pads with your hamstrings to full contraction and then slowly release.

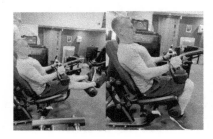

Seated or standing Calf Raise

Sit on a seated calf raise machine at your local gym. Position your feet on the footrest across the balls of your feet. Raise up on your toes to fully contract the calves. Now lower down below the level of the footrest to extend the calves completely. If you do not have a seated calf raise machine, you can do a standing calf raise using a kettlebell or dumbbell as seen here.

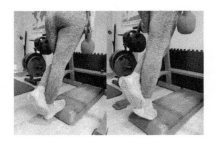

Alternative Dumbbell Reverse Lunges

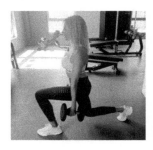

Using a mirror for this helps from a side view. Standing, take a large step backward with your right foot. Lower your hips so that your left thigh (front leg) becomes parallel to the floor so your left knee is directly above your ankle. Your right knee should be bent and in line with your torso pointing toward the floor with your heel lifted. Return to standing by pressing your left heel into the floor and bringing your right leg forward. Alternate legs.

Alternate Dumbbell Curl

Stand with a pair of dumbbells in your hands at your sides with palms facing your sides. Supinate your wrist as you curl the weight up to shoulder level. Be sure to keep your elbow in at your side and not to use momentum. Reverse the motion and repeat with the other arm.

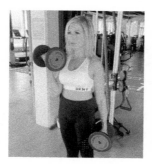

Decline Dumbbell Triceps Extension

Lie on a decline bench set to a 30 degree angle with a pair of dumbbells held above your head at full arm extension with your palms facing each other. Now bend at the elbows to bring the dumbbells down to the side of your head. Reverse the motion, being sure to keep your elbows in at your sides.

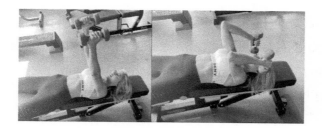

Barbell Wrist Curl

Sit on a bench with your knees together and a barbell in your hands. Place your forearms on your thighs so that your wrists and the weight are over your knees. Roll the barbell down your fingers to full extension and then curl the wrist up to full contraction. You can also do this with a dumbbell as seen below.

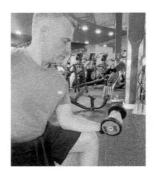

Barbell Hip Thrusts

Sit on the ground with a bench behind you. Keep your knees bent and hip width apart. Hold a barbell resting below your hips. Use a pad or towel for comfort. Lean back so your shoulder blades are on the bench and position the bar in the grove of your hips. Drive your hips up lifting the bar. At the top position your knees should be at 90°, with your body forming a straight line. Pause at the top of the lift and squeeze your glutes together, then lower your hips slowly. Start with no weight for higher reps.

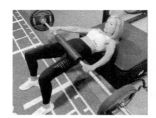